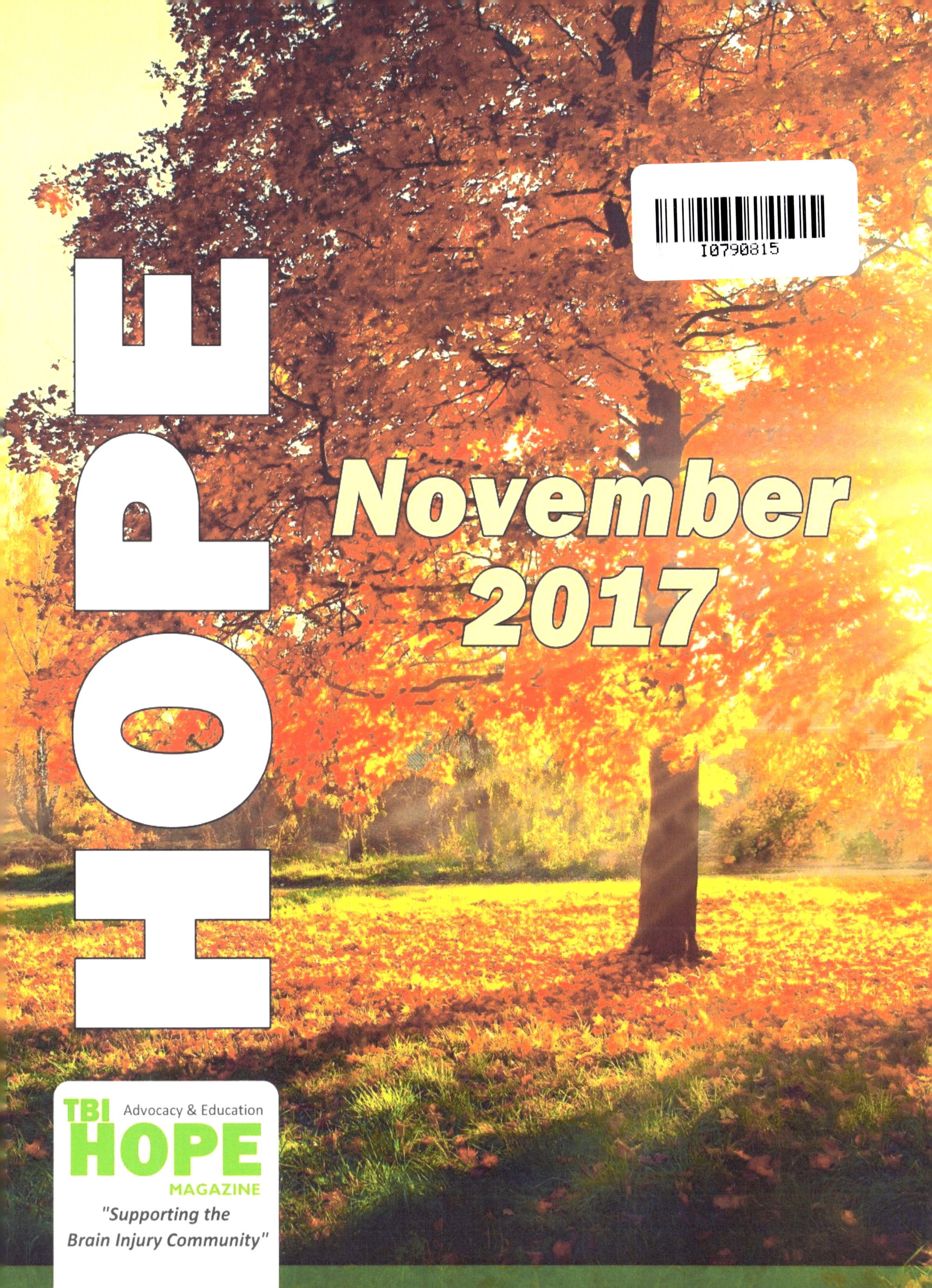
HOPE
November 2017
TBI
Advocacy & Education
HOPE
MAGAZINE
"Supporting the
Brain Injury Community"

Welcome

TBI HOPE MAGAZINE

Serving All Impacted by Brain Injury

November 2017

Publisher
David A. Grant

Editor
Sarah Grant

Contributing Writers
Cheryl Bigney
Nicole Charisi
Murray Dunlap
Debra Gorman
Ric Johnson
Tracie Massie
Norma Myers
Doug Prunier

Amazing Cartoonist
Patrick Brigham

*FREE subscriptions at
www.TBIHopeMagazine.com*

Welcome to the November 2017 issue of TBI HOPE Magazine!

As another year comes to a close, I like to look back over the past year to take stock of what has come to pass and look forward to how we can better serve the brain injury community.

As a publication, we have been able to touch thousands of lives every month. Both the print as well as digital versions of TBI Hope Magazine now have a worldwide readership.

A recent survey of our social community revealed some interesting facts. Eighty percent of our Facebook members are survivors, with the remaining 20% made up of family members, caregivers & professionals. We are truly a survivor-based community. Well over half of that community is over five years post-injury.

While these are interesting numbers, it does show that we need to find a better way to reach those newly injured. Those who have *"been there"* know that the first couple of years are the toughest.

As we move forward, we will be looking at new ways to serve those new to the brain injury community. If you have thoughts or suggestions, I would love to hear from you.

In the meantime, we will keep on "keeping on." It is our hope that you find some real hope in this month's issue.

Peace,

David A. Grant
Publisher

Contents

Gratitude makes sense of our past, brings peace for today, and creates a vision for tomorrow.

~Melody Beattie

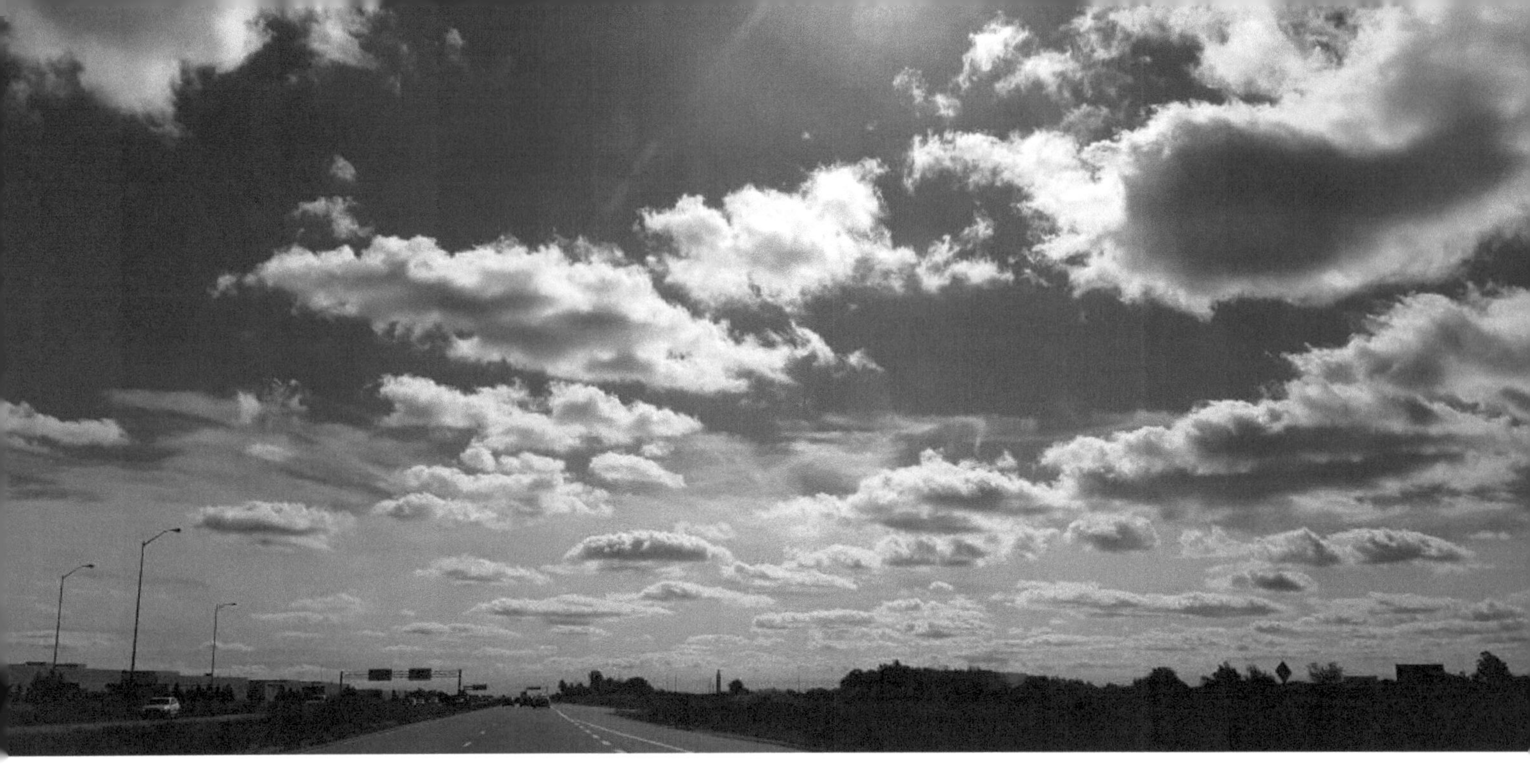

The Phone Call

By Tracie Massie

I was working, just like any other day, when my cell phone rang. On the other end was my sixteen-year-old son's high school vice-principal. His voice was soft and very sobering, unlike his usual joking and laughing. My first thought, like any mother would have, was what has he done now? As he started to speak, I knew this was not the usual, "your son is in trouble" phone call. The next words out of his mouth changed my life forever, "Tracie, Hank has had a car wreck and they are taking him to Grant Hospital."

I vaguely remember the thirty-mile drive to Columbus, Ohio. I do remember the weather that day was very strange. One minute the clouds were dark and threatening, the next minute the sun was shining beautifully. I tried to concentrate on the road and not the fact that if they were taking him thirty miles away, it had to be bad. I prayed endlessly, I bargained with God and I even questioned God - how He could take my husband ten years earlier, and now this.

> **I bargained with God and I even questioned God.**

He wants my son? I could not understand. I went from unbearable, mind-numbing fear, to anger and resentment in the blink of an eye. The road seemed to be endless. I know I was breaking the speed limit; the hum of the V-6 cruising down the road was at a constant rate. I felt like I was in slow motion, on a treadmill and not making any progress. Was I ever going to get there?

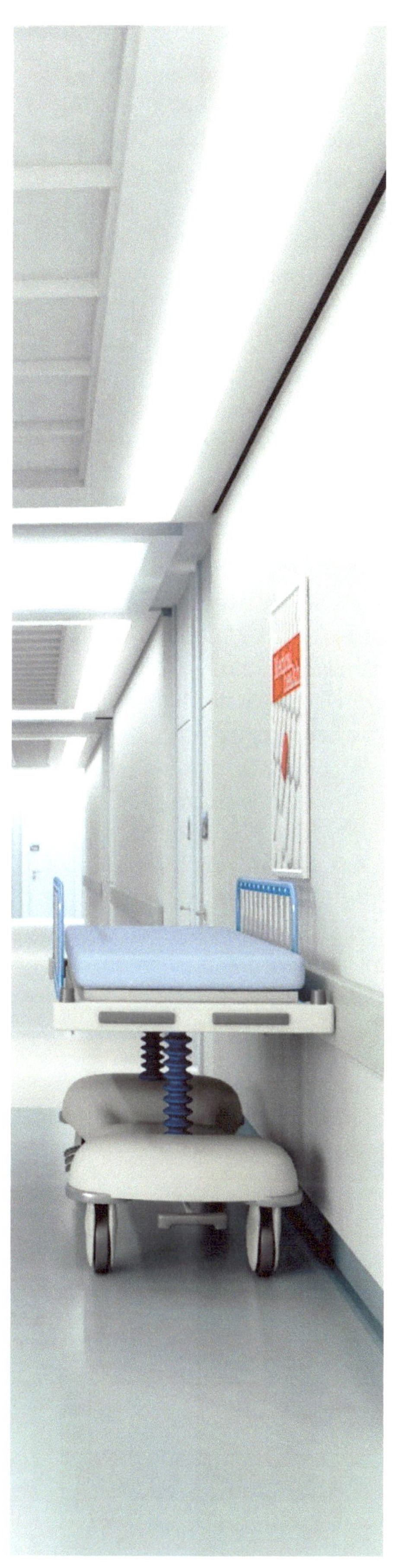

Finally, I pulled into the parking garage. The walk to the emergency room took forever. I walked in to an arena of orderly chaos with nurses, crying children, and various other staff members everywhere. A motherly looking woman asked if she could help me. In the strongest voice I could muster, I told her my son had been brought into the emergency room. At that point she made a quick phone call and located my son. I remember hearing her say that they were taking him to surgery. I told her Hank could not go until I saw him. She was trying to explain to me why I could not see him, when the head of the trauma department came in and told her to call upstairs and hold my son outside of the operating room.

The doctor took me through the doors straight to the operating area so I could see my son before he went in. I will never forget that sight as long as I live. It was a very sterile-feeling area and my son was laying there motionless. I remember thinking, "there is nothing wrong, there isn't any blood." The only thing that I noticed about him was his chest seemed twice as thick. Little did I know that all of his internal organs were in his chest cavity.

After giving him a kiss and telling him that I loved him, they took him away. The nurse guided me to a small, quiet room where she said I could wait for the surgeon, and by this time my whole family had arrived. I was still in a fog and it seemed as though I was watching all of this from above, like an out of body experience.

After what seemed like an eternity, the surgeon walked in. God had spared my son. He explained all of his internal injuries, along with a traumatic brain injury. The doctor was hopeful concerning his recovery and tried to prepare me for what I would see when I went into the room. I had worked in the healthcare field for most of my adult life, but that did not even prepare me for what I saw. In a small cubicle my son was hooked to every machine imaginable, IV's with four different bags attached, heart monitor, pump for the chest tube, bag for the G-tube, catheter and ventilator. My heart sank. This could not be my baby. The mass of wires, monitors, and beeping machines was not my baby. After nine weeks in the hospital, we went home.

He was not the young man I said good-bye to that October morning, but he was alive. It has been eleven years and if you did not know him before, you would not know a thing happened until you saw the scars. He has a scar stretching from his sternum to his pelvic area, with several quarter sized areas from the incision dehiscing. A scar from his trachea, G-tube, two chest tubes, and a cut on his elbow that is about four inches long.

It has been eleven years since his accident. Hank will never be the same. The young man that left that Wednesday morning for school never returned. I still love him with all my heart. The Hank that left that day was patient, big hearted, easy going, with a great sense of humor. The accident left him with depression, arthritis, emphysema, asthma, his left diaphragm does not work and he has narrowing of the trachea. With all of this, I still thank God every day for sparing his life. We have our battles, because everything I taught him as he was growing up left him when the semi hit the car. I just pray God continues to intervene between the two of us so we can get through the days ahead.

Meet Tracie Massie

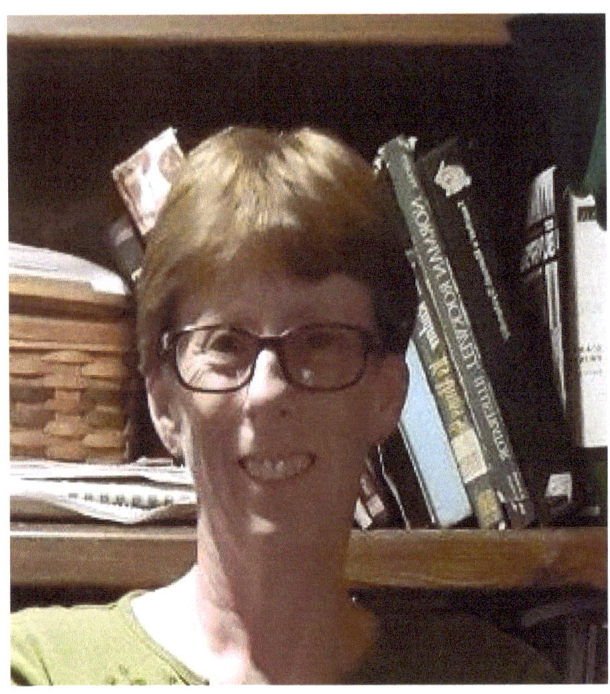

Tracie Writes…
"I live in Darbyville, Ohio and work for our local school as teacher's aide for special needs and IEP students. I am the mother of a TBI survivor. My son's TBI occurred when he pulled out in front of a semi in 2006. He was in a coma for three weeks at Grant Medical Center and spent six weeks in rehab at Nationwide Children's Hospital. He has suffered two more TBI's since - one due to another car accident and the third happened when he was jumped by three people and kicked in the head repeatedly. I worked in the healthcare field almost my entire adult life, which was a huge help when it came to caring for my son after the accident. But I really believe his TBI prepared me for the job I have now working with special needs children. I have found that it has awakened a passion inside me for helping do all I can for them and be an advocate for them when needed."

Living With Hope

By Patrick Brigham

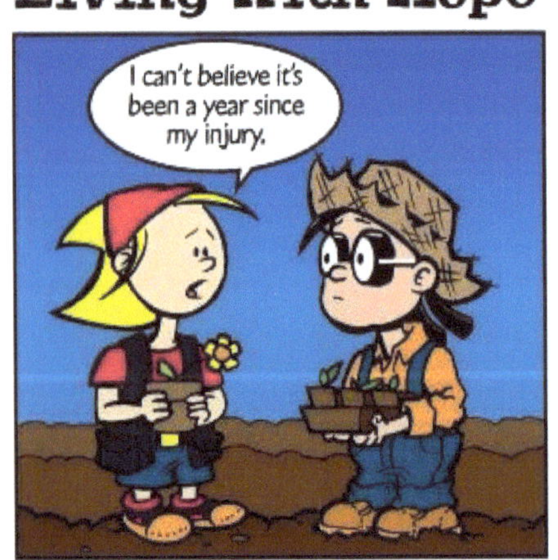

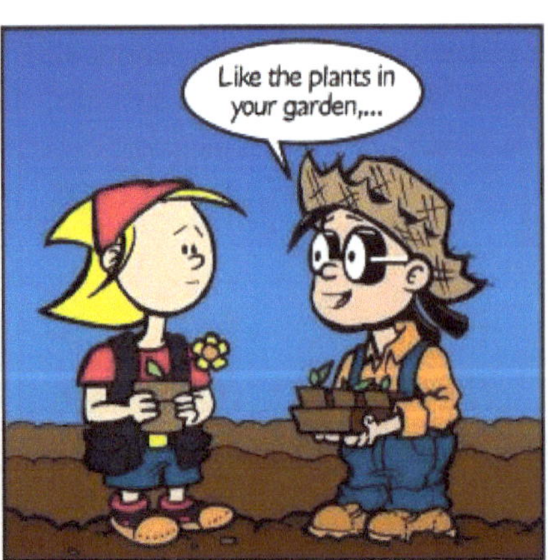

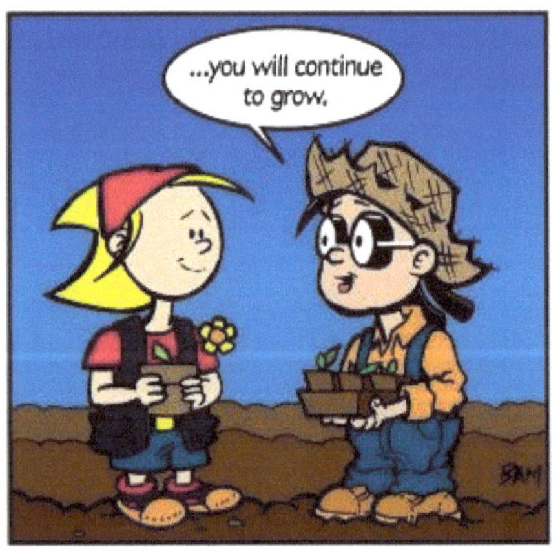

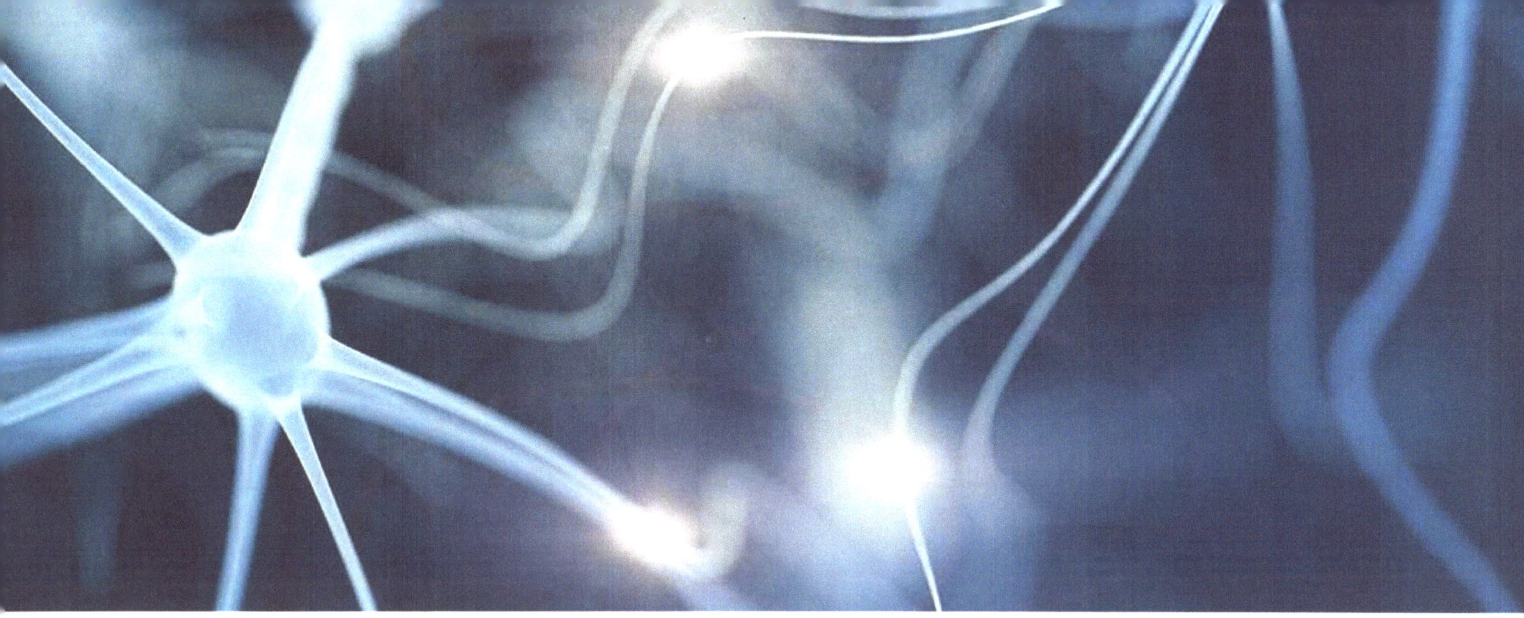

Thank you, Mr. Brain!

By Ric Johnson

It's 7:00 AM and I'm awake and ready for today. Actually, pretty much ready for any day. It is all because of you, so let me say thanks, Mr. Brain. Thanks for giving me my new life.

October 18, 2003, was a day we did not see coming. After falling off a ladder while cleaning gutters on my house, I broke you, but you did not give up. I was in a coma. Craniology surgery removed a bone from my skull. I woke up a month later and had to relearn to do everyday tasks. These were tasks that my parents taught me before I was five years old. Thank you for remembering many important things with your long-time working memory.

You made it through speech and occupational therapy almost without missing a beat. It did take a year before I graduated from therapy, but you found new paths, new connections, and new memories. It is hard to know where I would be without you.

> **I woke up a month later and had to relearn to do everyday tasks.**

I also want to make sure to say that I love the instructions you give me every day. It is your voice allowing me to have good days instead of bad days. Each day you tell me to see the past, or where we were a day or a week, or a month ago. Each day you tell me to see the present and see what tasks or appointments are scheduled. Each day you tell me not to wonder about the future. You already know that I have wondered about the future, but now I know it is a worthless cause. Why is thinking about the future worthless? Because of you Mr. Brain, because of you.

You have made wonderful progress, so much more than what my family was told and more than what I ever thought possible during that first year. Not every day is a good day. Short-term memory comes and goes, aphasia comes and goes, but overall most days are good days.

Your ability to see, to plan, and to execute chores and tasks amazes me. As long as I follow your directions about eating, drinking, sleeping, and caring about my body, I am sure that you won't let me down. You needed to be both my pre-injury brain and my post-injury brain at the same time, to let me go forward. You did and you continue to guide my actions.

I have asked you to allow me to be a good husband, father and grandfather. I have asked you to help with short-term memory so I can still be employed. I have asked you to tell me when it is time for a nap. I have asked you to let me believe in myself. You have never failed me.

Instead of being a silent partner, you are my doctor and minister. Instead of being a walking victim, you gave me a vision and voice. Instead of being overwhelmed by life in general, you gave me the ability to release frustration for situations I cannot control.

Every day after waking up, I open my eyes and say "Hello brain, thanks for giving me yesterday and letting me look forward to today." I may not stop asking for favors so I am sending this note to say "Thank You, Mr. Brain, for all you have done!"

Meet Ric Johnson

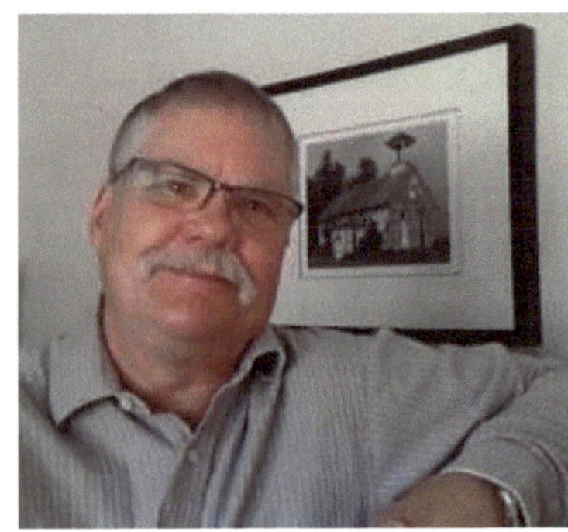

Ric Johnson is a husband, father, grandfather and a traumatic brain injury survivor from just over 13 years.

Ric is also a member of the Speaker Bureau for the Minnesota Brain Injury Alliance, and facilitator for The Courage Kenny Brain Injury Support Group.

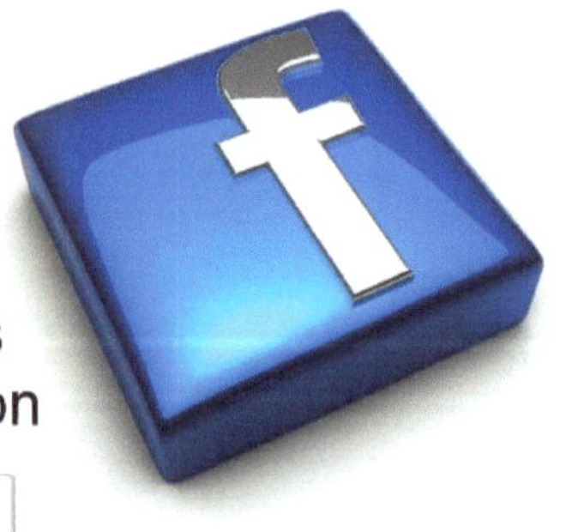

Finding Senior Housing can be complex, but it doesn't have to be.

Call A Place for Mom. Our Advisors are trusted, local experts who can help you understand your options. Since 2000, we've helped over one million families find senior living solutions that meet their unique needs.

"You can trust **A Place for Mom** to help you."

– Joan Lunden

a Place *for* Mom.

A Free Service for Families.
Call: (844) 578-9504

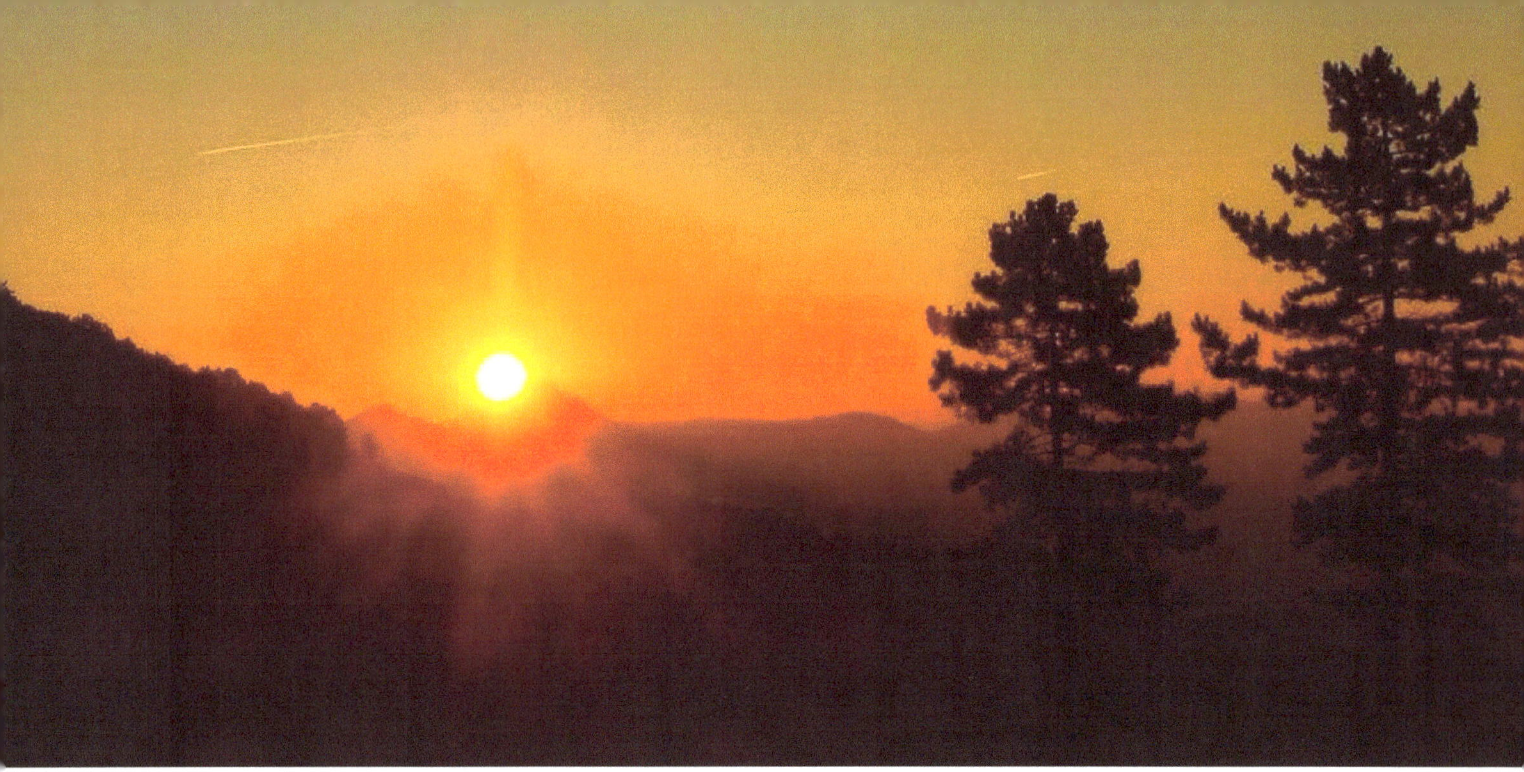

Firsts
By Norma Myers

Upon hearing the words, "*You are going to be a Mom*," I immediately started counting down! There is the due date, followed by the infamous recording of every first! First word, first step…you remember! As time marches on, in what felt like a blink of an eye, we were parents of young adults. *Our* plan included helping our sons through their "normal" firsts: high school, college, career, marriage, and children. Nowhere on our "*normal*" firsts list was finding ourselves sitting by our 22-year-old son's hospital bed praying that he would live.

Our only children Aaron and Steven were involved in a car accident in August 2012. Upon hearing that our son Steven sustained a severe Traumatic Brain Injury (TBI), our focus was on his survival, not on what the life changing diagnosis held for us. Ashamedly, I admit that until TBI happened to us, I was not educated enough to understand that we would be going down the path of awaiting firsts all over again. Fragile life and death firsts. Life, as in, *will Steven survive?* And death: *our firstborn son, Aaron, didn't survive.* Hearing Steven's diagnosis coupled with Aaron's death, blew our hearts, minds, and bodies with shocking *firsts* we could never have imagined. This kind of catastrophic news happens in movies, not in our ordinary life!

When asking medical staff about Steven's outcome, the unequivocal response was, "Every Brain Injury is different. It's too early to tell." We weren't asking about possible deficits; we only ***needed*** to know if

Steven was going to wake up. What if I never heard Steven call me Mom again? The thought caused my heart to skip a beat and my brain to radically recalculate as I hoped for a different outcome, and this hope sprang against the reality that *I would never hear **Aaron** call me Mom again*. How could I accept such a hard calculation? I didn't. Instead, I rebooted and shifted my focus to Steven. He needed me, and I needed him!

I have learned that being in shock can be a lifesaver. For me, it provided a protective coating of armor around my heart, the kind of protection necessary to prepare me to see Steven through TBI firsts—the kind of firsts that brought a different level of joy to my heart and tears to my eyes, versus newborn firsts.

The most grueling first as parents happened several weeks after the accident when Steven's doctor gave his approval to deliver the news of Aaron's death to Steven. We were not equipped to speak those horrible words any more than Steven's ears were prepared to hear, his fragile brain to process or his tender heart to receive. In the stillness of that room at the Shepherd Center with my husband by my side offering a sense of strength, I held Steven's hand, and as my voice threatened to leave me, I whispered to our son, "Steven, you have been asking about Aaron and why your brother hasn't been to visit you.

I need you to listen to me. We need to talk to you about the accident. I know you don't remember, but Aaron was with you. I don't know how to tell you honey, but Aaron didn't make it…he's gone."

Without an audible response, Steven's grueling expression told me that his heart was breaking in a way that he would relive for the rest of his life. The kind of heartbreak that reminded us once again that we would never be the same.

Unless you have been touched by the messy world of TBI, doubled with losing a child you aren't expected to understand that becoming Steven's caregiver saved my life. The pain from losing Aaron was excruciating enough to cut off my life sustaining air supply. I will always remember the shock of seeing Steven in the Emergency Room. The medical professionals tried to prepare us, but despite the most prestigious credentials, how does one do that? They can't! As soon as I saw my unrecognizable son, I knew that I had a life sustaining purpose. Knowing that my son needed me gave strength to my buckling knees. No matter how crippling the agony of our reality, there was no way I was going to miss witnessing Steven's miraculous comeback. What a show it has been, especially from the front row seat!

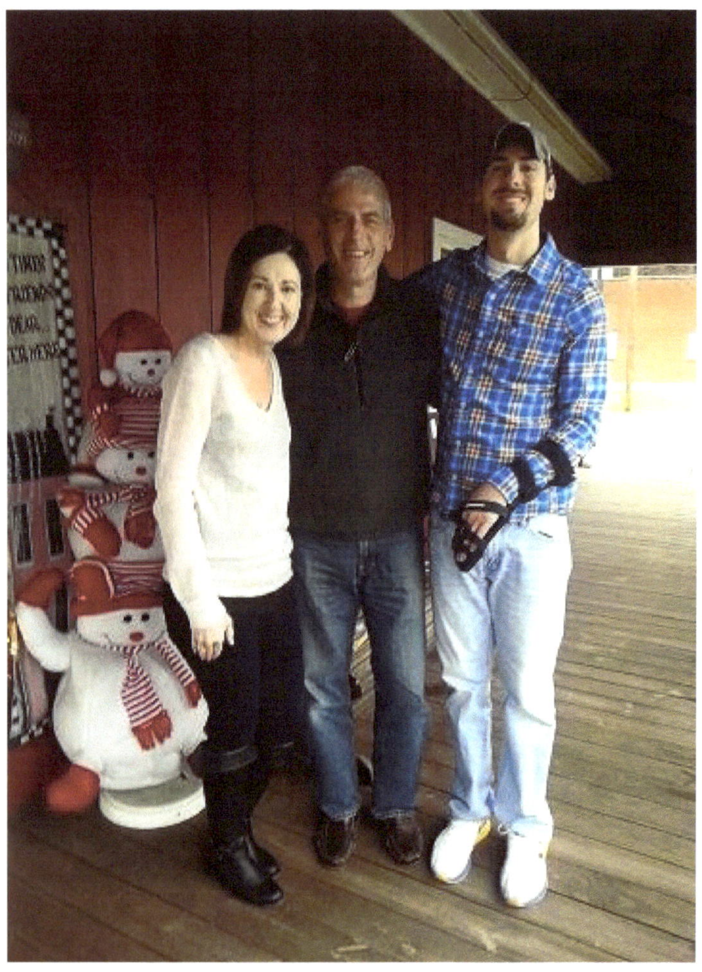

This past August marked five years since our lives changed. Steven has bravely fought his way through recovery. He conquered every first with the ferociousness of a young man who ultimately knew his parent's survival depended upon his own. Upon hearing the devastating news of Aaron not surviving, Steven made a determined promise of not giving up to his brother. He has gone above and beyond to keep his word.

We have celebrated Steven returning to college, hiking his favorite trail, getting back behind the wheel, becoming employed and, most recently, swimming in the ocean for the first time since before the accident. During our recent family vacation in the Outer Banks of NC; where our sons spent countless hours together, I watched Steven approach the ocean with confidence. For selfish "needing to protect my son" reasons, I offered Steven every excuse to stay out of the ocean. Steven smiled, offered reassuring words that did not reach my ears, and he enjoyed the ocean. Meanwhile, I stood frozen in the sand, praying to God to protect our son. As Steven enjoyed the healing ocean waves, my heart was being assaulted by emotional waves of the relentless WHAT IF's? I was proud of Steven for stepping out of his comfort zone, ultimately causing me to do the same. I know he was more than ready to be in the ocean long before that moment. More times than I have been aware, he has been mindful and protective of his mom's fragile heart.

Our journey has taught us many lessons. Among the top of the list is not expecting others to understand what we are going through. People don't know what to say. It's okay. We don't always know what to say. We are repeatedly told that we are admired. Often, those words are followed by an awkward hesitation. Allow me to finish the sentence, "***We admire you, but we don't want to be you!***" Agreed! No parent should outlive their child, doubled with navigating the unpredictable diagnosis of TBI.

Our desire is, instead of being parents that remind you of your worst nightmare, may we be a reminder that when trauma strikes you won't feel prepared! You will freak out! You will cry until you think you can't possibly produce one more tear. You will scream at the top of your lungs, "I can't do, this!" But, there is good news! God designed us to be protectors of our children. In times of need, we dig deeper physically, emotionally & spiritually than we think is humanly possible to be present for our children, our husband, our family, and friends. You can survive even when you think there is no possible way!

Through our journey, we have become super-glued as a family with understanding and respect of how the unwelcomed knock on our door has and will continue to affect each of us differently. There's no "one size fits all!" We acknowledge that our family, friends, and community have been affected. We are blessed by the ones that have stayed and understand when others couldn't.

The welcome back mat is always out!

My heart hurts for everyone who has been touched by our journey. We understand the pain you have felt. On the days when our emotional tanks were empty, we found strength from your love and support. We know there will be more firsts, some welcomed, others unwelcomed. I admire Steven for not allowing TBI to define or limit him. I have lessons to learn from him as I often find myself feeling defined by my losses. I am told that these feelings go along with the identity crisis that is experienced with a life-changing event. This certainly meets the "life change" event criteria.

It is my choice each day to decide if I will drown in my losses or be thankful for what's right in front of me, I can learn and grow from both. Despite what happens to me, ultimately, I decide whether I dwell in the ugly or live in the here and now, in which, despite all losses, beauty can be found. It is in the dark times that the light of family, friends, and community shines the brightest.

Instead of getting lost in the dizzying doom and gloom of my circumstances, I strive to rise above, be present for my family and be willing to help others that are hurting. Daily, I will continue to honor Aaron's memory, celebrate Steven's life, and thank God for the blessings that are right in front of me.

Meet Norma Myers

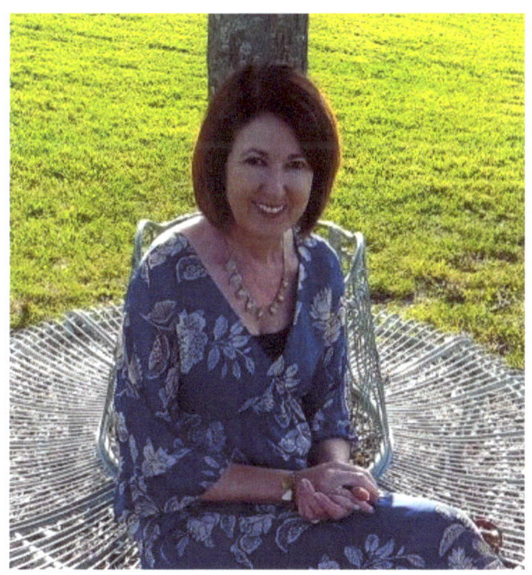

Norma and her husband Carlan spend much of their time supporting their son Steven as he continues on his road to recovery. Norma is an advocate for those recovering from traumatic brain injury.

Her written work has been featured on Brainline.org, a multi-media website that serves the brain injury community. Her family continues to heal.

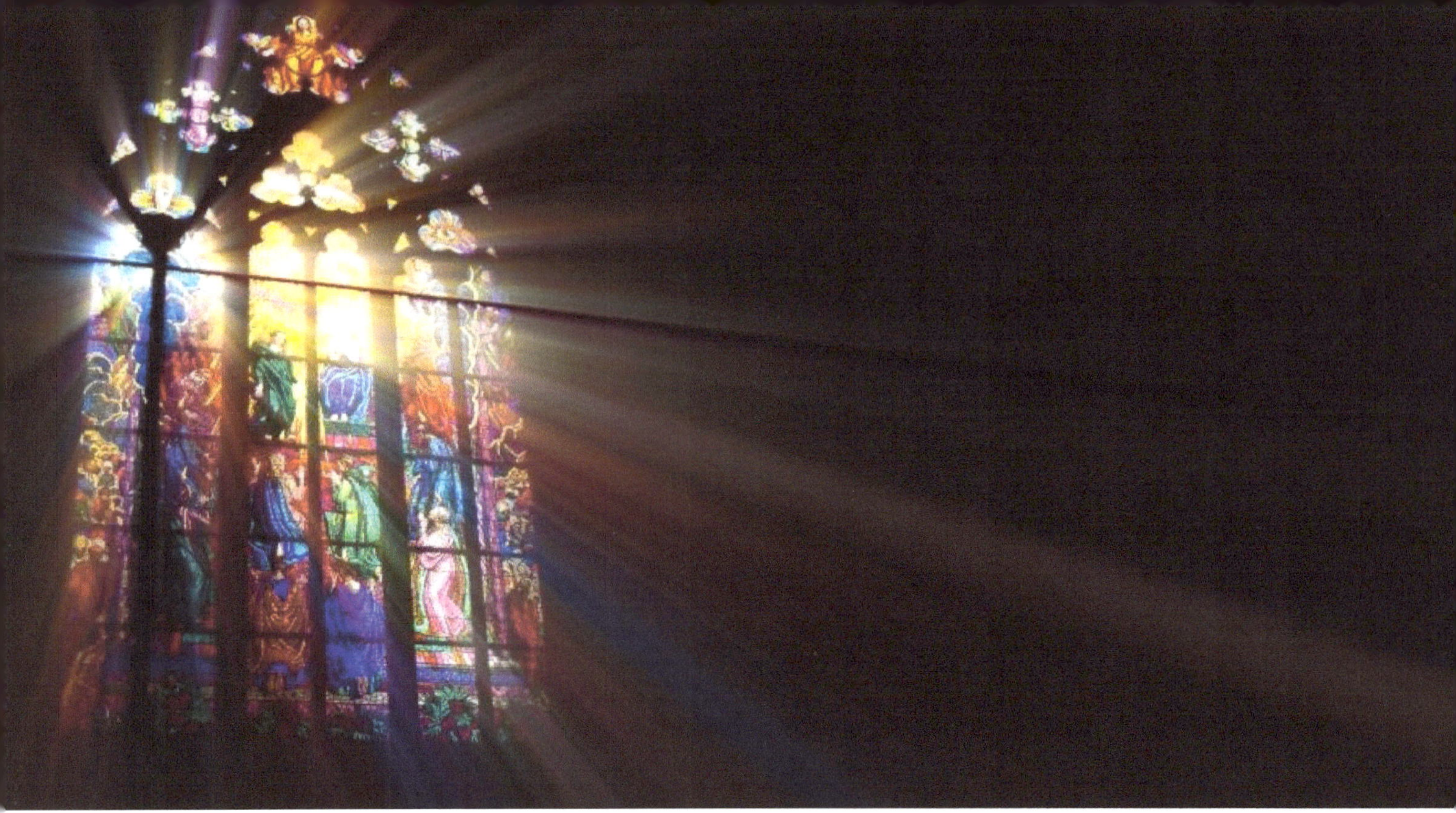

On my Knees

By Murray Dunlap

Today, I am on my knees and thanking God I am alive. Yesterday, I was driving on my street when I was crushed by bending metal and broken glass. But today, I am on my knees.

At 34, a nice man missed a red light and everything about my life changed. I have a traumatic brain injury. I was a married writer about to start a new career as an English teacher. Our marriage could not survive the confusion and amnesia. When asked, I did not know I was married. After more doctors and therapy than I can remember, I am a writer again with a new book of poetry called *Proof*. I have met, fallen in love with, and married an Episcopal priest. I am not the man I once was. I am better.

> # I am not the man I once was. I am better.

The old Murray died on June 7, 2008, in a car wreck, so I've been forced to reinvent myself. I spent close to three months in a coma, followed by several months in a wheelchair (I can't remember how long due to amnesia – it seemed like forever) and many more using a walker. I had three fractures in my pelvis, a broken clavicle, nine sutures in my head, and five stitches in my ear. I also had fourth nerve palsy (double vision), which required surgery. I lost most all of my ability to stay balanced. Just walking can be hard. Without a railing, stairs are not possible. Worst of all, I have a traumatic brain injury, which is a complex injury with a broad spectrum of symptoms and disabilities. I was forced to relearn to walk, to drive, to stop speaking with a slur and crooked eyebrows, and the worst thing (to me personally), a smile that drooped on one side of my mouth. I put myself back together and now jog most days (as a former distance runner, this is now a slow, strange gait, but I'm out there!) I lost the 50 pounds I gained in my wheelchair and walker days, and gave up alcohol. I speak clearly with very little slur, my eyebrows line up, and my smile is finally straight. I finished my second book, called "Fires," and wrote a book of poetry called "Proof," which is forthcoming. Around the next corner, my sister-in-law

introduced me to the love of my life – an Episcopal priest named Mary Balfour.

Now, for a few of the ways my life was made strange by a brain injury. I will spare you my misadventures with teeth, memory, balance and online dating. Instead, I need to share about my ability to run.

One way that my life has been strange, more frustrating really, is running. I had been an avid distance runner and one day measured 26 miles in my car, and then I ran it, just to see if I could. In those days, I could.

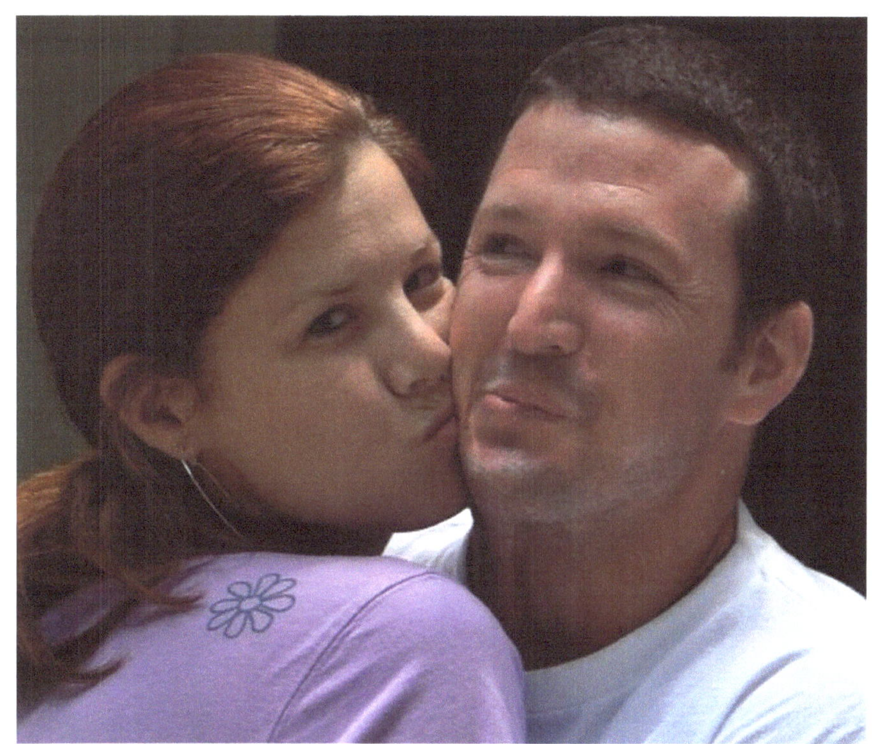

Since the wheelchair, my 'jogs' have been a strange walking-thing. I even tried to convince myself that I was, in fact, actually jogging. I was not. But, considering I lost the 50 pounds I gained in my wheelchair and walker days, so what if I look silly? It has been difficult to adjust to people seeing my strange gait and stopping to ask me if I am ok. I have learned that it is only out of care that they do this, and not fascination at how strange I appear. I admit that I am proud of what I have done, and very excited that I no longer need new pants. In fact, I was third in my age group in a 5K last year. Now, there may well have only been three runners my age, but dammit, I was out there trying.

I had gone from living in my mother's garage because of unrelenting confusion in my mid 30's, to asking the bishop for permission to marry my wife – an Episcopal priest, in my early 40's, and rejoining my family and the Episcopal Church. I am happy to add that, of course because she is now my wife, I was given permission to propose, and I am now on a first name basis with the Alabama Bishop and we do not shake hands, we hug.

Sleep is a thing we all take for granted, but has been hell on earth for me. Following the wreck, I was on much, much medication. So much, that the people surrounding me had trouble telling me what to take, and when. I had reached 18 pills a day. So, this was made easier by giving me a pile of pills with each meal. The problem was that the number of doctors and different pills left mixing medicine impossible to watch. Who knows what was actually going on, but the result was that I was falling asleep at about seven o'clock in the evening. This went on for long enough that my body got used to going to sleep at this hour, and I have been forced to make slow adjustments of going to sleep a bit later each month or so to reach a normal nightly schedule.

I need to say that this is a guess on my part. I have no idea how my sleep patterns were moved to such strange hours. What I do know is that I have spent the night at a hospital in Mobile, Alabama, and one in Birmingham to let doctors watch me sleep. At Grandview hospital in Birmingham they discovered my sleep apnea. I have no idea if this was caused by the wreck, but what I do know is that I stop breathing seven times an hour when I sleep. Stop breathing? And seven times an hour? That's not restful at all.

But, with this knowledge, I have been given a c-pap machine that I wear at night. A c-pap is a machine that generates a solid flow of air into my nose all night long, and thus, has given me the best sleep I have had since the wreck. I wake with the ability to think clearly and have learned to trust myself.

In a wonderful turn, I have a new book coming out soon called Proof. Two years ago, my wife and I hatched a plan for me to write a poem a day for 90 days. It was my job for the summer. After accomplishing this goal, I kept going until I had 130 poems and rewritten most of the 90. It gave me great satisfaction to discover I had written a book.

From the very deepest, suicidal despair, to the glorious joy of true love, my life has started making sense again.

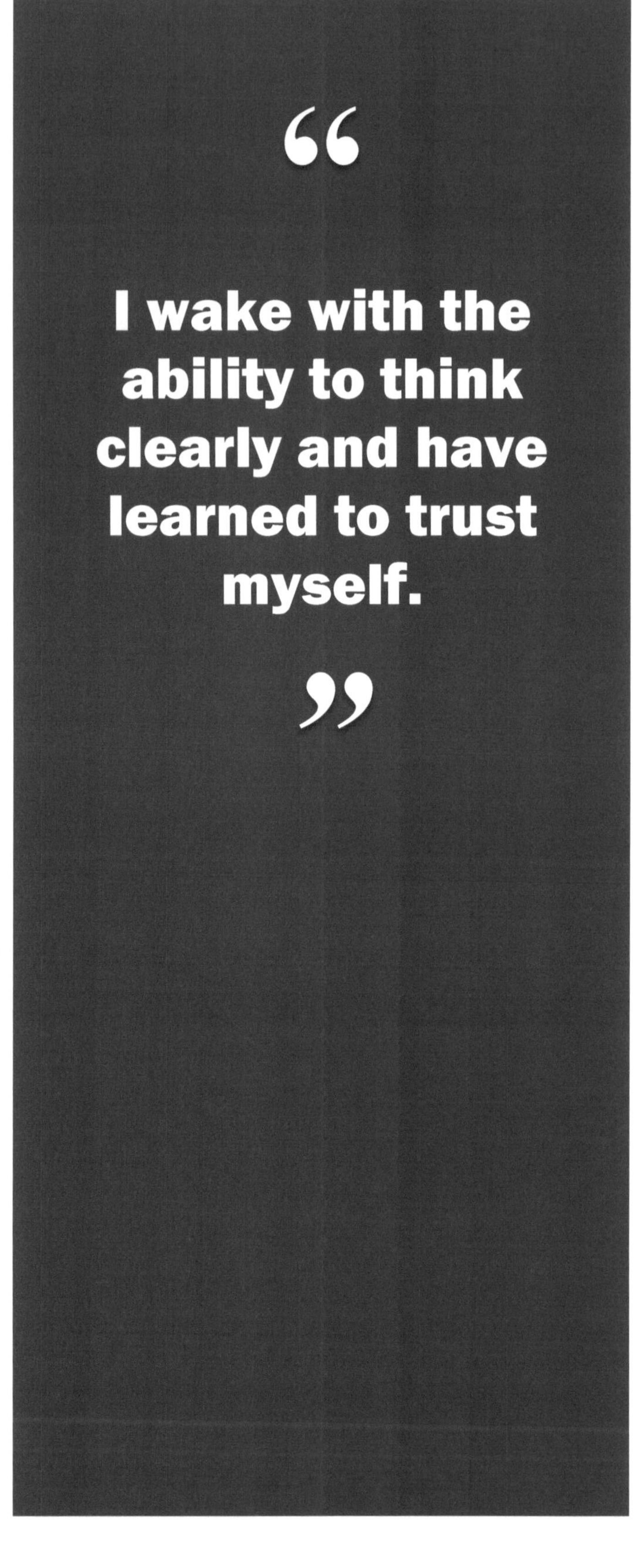

I had lost track of God and resented my arduous journey, but I have learned that the wreck was not God's plan. My recovery and meeting the love of my life was. A new Murray says, "From nearly dead to newlywed, I'm making the most of it. Life is hard but, never give up!"

With a brain injury, I am unable to work like most people. So, I wrote a few books, married a priest, found God, and learned to believe in myself. Yesterday was more pain and suffering than a person should ever be forced to endure, but today, I am on my knees, and thanking God I am alive!

Meet Murray Dunlap

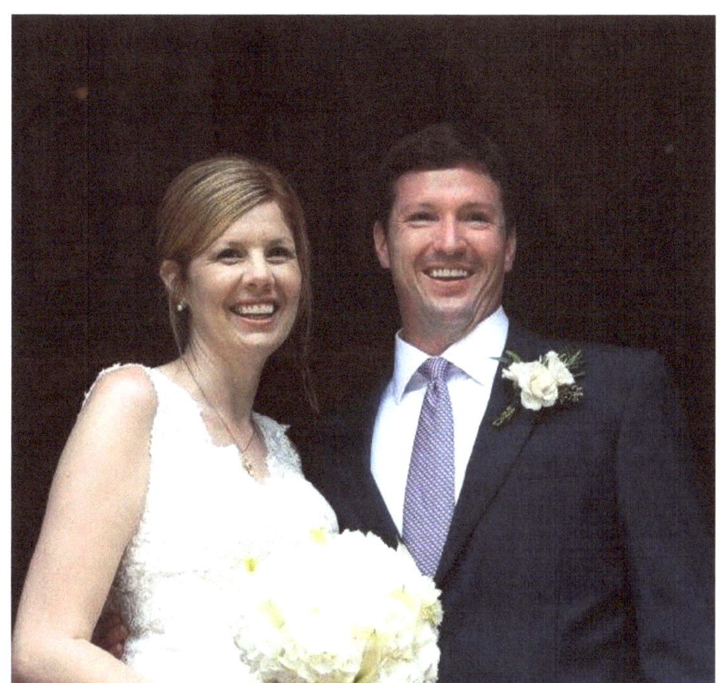

Murray Dunlap's work has appeared in numerous magazines and journals. His stories have been nominated for the Pushcart Prize three times, as well as to Best New American Voices. The story 'Race Day' was a finalist for the American Fiction Short Story award, 2014.

Dunlap has an MA in creative writing from U.C. Davis. The extraordinary individuals Pam Houston, Michael Knight, and Fred Ashe taught him the art of writing.

Murray is a writer again with a new book coming out called Proof. He met, fell in love with, and married an Episcopal priest. He shares, "I am not the man I once was. I am better."

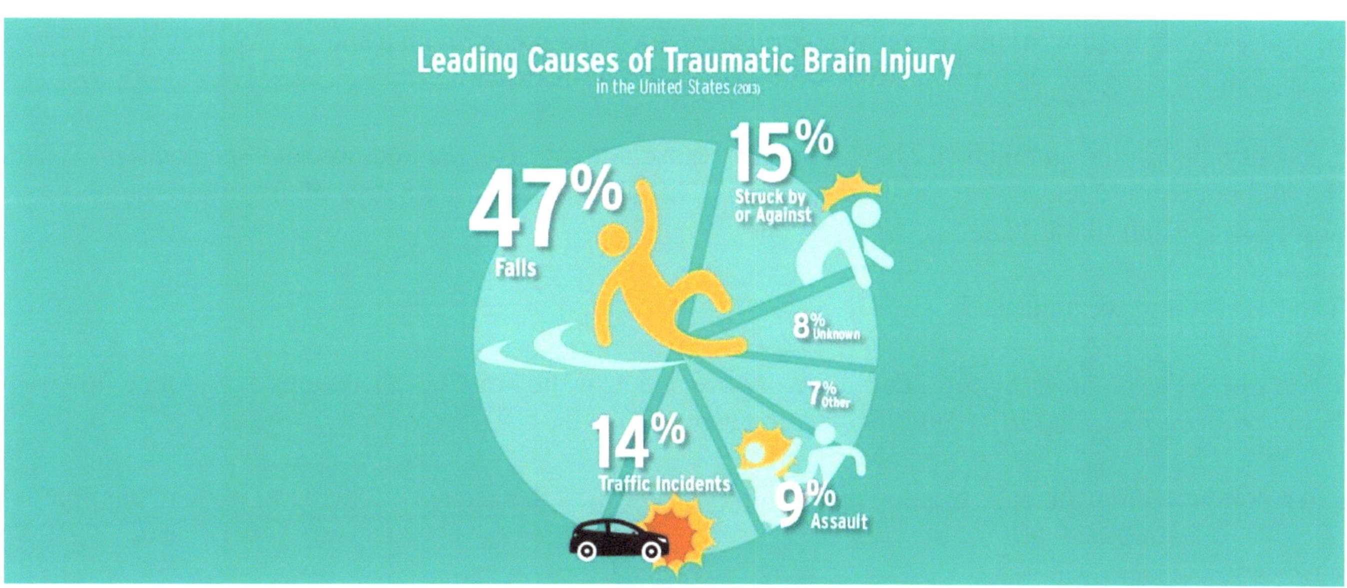

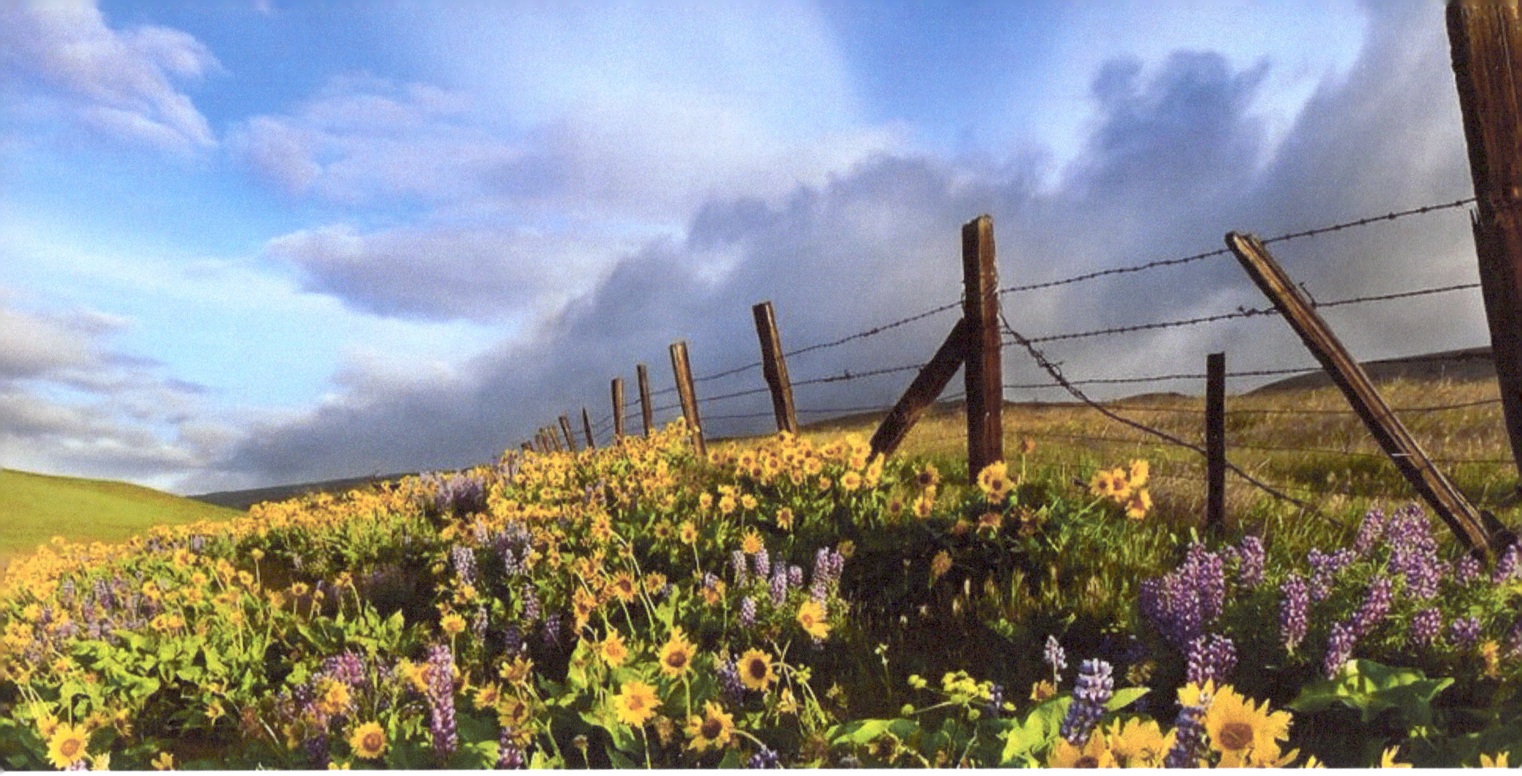

Memory is Life

By Cheryl Bigney

In the 1980s movie *Regarding Henry,* Harrison Ford was a successful lawyer who was shot in the head at the corner store. After his injury, he fell into a coma, suffered anoxia, and he finally woke up - but with the mind of a child. He had to learn to walk again, to talk again, and to read again. This is my story exactly.

In my case, my head went into the key ignition after a T-bone collision on a snowy day. It was the day after Thanksgiving in 1987. I was a thirteen-year-old girl at the time.

I actually died in the ambulance. They could not resuscitate me. The paramedics tried the paddles. When that did not work, decided to try manual pressure. This is when I left my body. While still in the ambulance, it felt like I floated above everyone.

Then everything went black.

It felt like I was on an escalator. I could see my life and hear the noises of the events as I looked down below. It brings to mind *It's a Small World,* at Disney World.

I just continued to walk up. I was so happy with no other thoughts except excitement, joy and happiness.

A little blond boy, about the age of five, came up to me and began to walk with me. He grabbed my hand. I glanced at him, but he did not look up at me. I kept walking. We both stopped. I saw the light, that so many others see and a voice said, "It's not time yet."

The next thing I knew, I was in a hospital bed, trying to answer the nurse when she asked me what flavor shake I wanted. I finally said, "Chocolate".

After waking up from a ten-day coma, I was unable to recognize my mom or my dad. I cried each time they left the room. I was able to learn things quickly. I learned to walk again. I could read words on the doors.

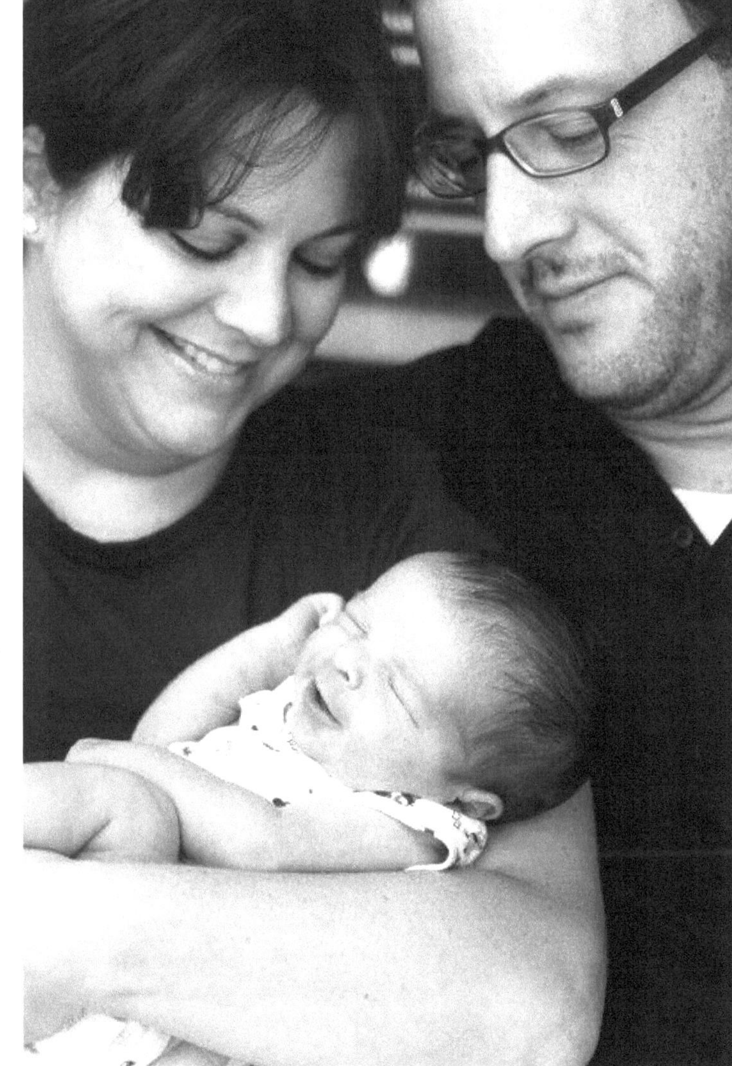

What I lost, however, was everything about me. Like a child, I had no self-image, no ego, and no identity. That is where my real recovery, which took the next twenty-five years, took place.

Somehow in that abyss, I knew I had had the perfect childhood, and that childhood was gone forever. I forgot all the people and had lost all the memories. I felt sad. I could not talk yet and had no way to explain this. I had to deal with the loss of virtually everything.

Next came returning to school. This was like a social boot camp. It was as tough as nails and probably got me back as far as I am today. I was confused, overwhelmed, and just hated myself because I had no explanation of why my life was so horrible. I ended up trying to kill myself.

After a heartfelt prayer, my answer finally came. In my sophomore year, a girl transferred to our school. I literally just became her. I took on her personality and her self-image. I had to be someone. She unknowingly saved my life.

Then came Senior Dinner with lifelong childhood friends who knew me long before the accident. They saw what happened to me. They awarded me Class Airhead, Most Likely to Get Lost in the Halls, and Most Likely to Be Found on a Milk Carton.

Today, I am forty-five and happily married with two kids. I go from pretending it never happened (such a relief), to trying to redo the memories, to hating the accident and everything about it (very empowering), to trying to see it as just something that happened a long time ago (this doesn't work), to just feeling like I'm back now. It's complicated.

I am doing this so I can find the best consciousness to live in, because these recovery memories are like war memories, and to let them stay in your life is almost like allowing myself to be ruined by them. Even today, I still go back and forth, just trying to find a way to deal with the past, so it doesn't keep diminishing my present happiness.

Memory is life. Friends are life. Self-image is life. That is why we are all here, sharing our stories.

Meet Cheryl Bigney

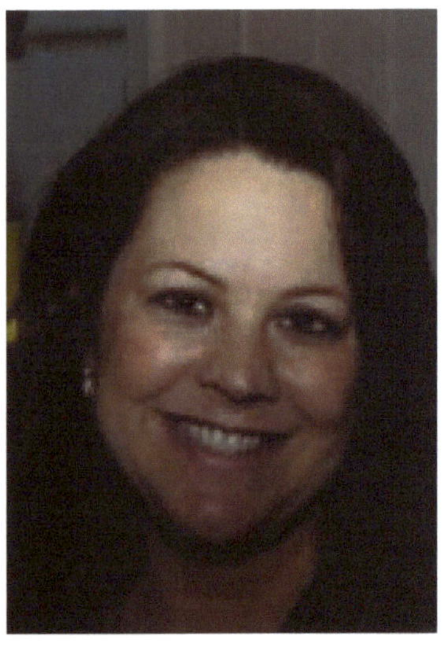

Cheryl Bigney is a stay-at-home mom and freelance writer in the Chicago suburbs. She studied Journalism and Psychology at Indiana University-Bloomington, and had a career as an advertising copywriter.

After a whole life of acting as if nothing really happened, Cheryl is ready to share her story. With her recovery, she offers meaningful insights into TBI recovery and personality recovery, and hopes she can help others also on this arduous journey.

I always like to look on the optimistic side of life, but I am realistic enough to know that life is a complex matter.

~Walt Disney

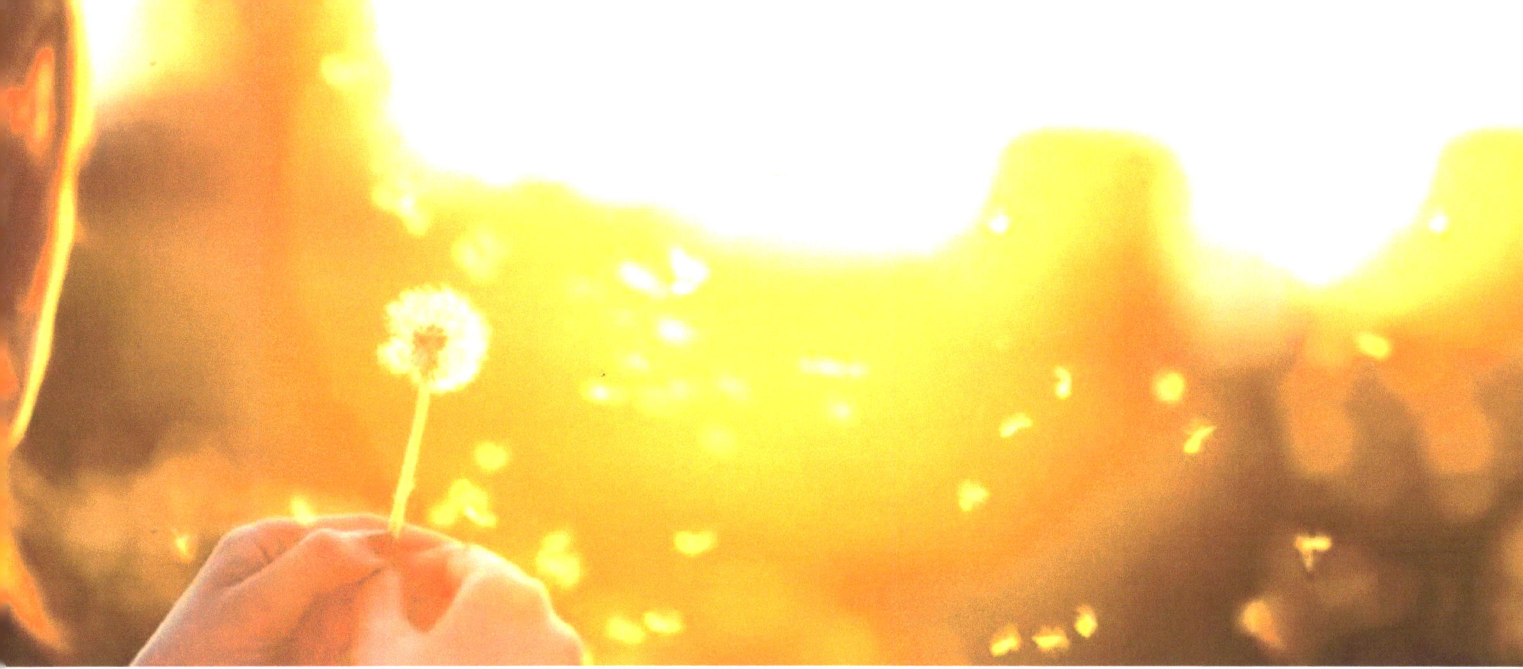

Happiness is a Choice

By Debra Gorman

It was six years ago, August 20, 2011. (You never forget the date, do you?) My brain started to hemorrhage from a condition I was apparently born with, called a Cavernous Angioma, on my brainstem. It was considered inoperable and the bleeding in my brain led to a stroke. My life hung in the balance for several days, but survive, I did.

I worked very hard those first years at all sorts of therapy. I was absolutely determined I would return to my former state of being and recover my past abilities. Otherwise, I didn't know how I would face life. I didn't know if I *could* face life. I was fifty-six years old at the time of the event. I had spent nearly a lifetime being one way.

> **I was absolutely determined I would return to my former state of being and recover my past abilities.**

Time passed and I struggled. I applied tremendous effort for improvements that either didn't come, or were so minor I didn't want to count them. It was slowly becoming clear to me that I was never going to be who I was before.

So, I turned my efforts to accepting my new limitations. I believed the key to my acceptance was to carve out a satisfying life around the interests and abilities I had always had, approaching them in a new way; a way more accessible to me now, as my methods had to be different from before.

I missed my old life terribly. Formerly, I had built my life around a fairly new marriage, other relationships, my career, hobbies and interests. For example, I had been a long distance runner, a backpacker, bodybuilder, and long distance cyclist. I was also a nurse, a do-it-yourselfer, a decorator, traveler, actor, and director. I took pride in all those things. They were all activities that I felt somehow defined me, but which were out of the question for me now. Recently, however, I recalled that while backpacking many years ago I decided that when I became old and feeble, I could take up canoeing and do some primitive camping on various islands. Perhaps I would even take up fishing, which I had pursued and enjoyed in my twenties. When I made that future decision, I had in mind my eighties, but now might be a good time to explore those options.

I also enjoy writing and have more time for it. More time is needed because I must peck at the keyboard with the thumb and forefinger of my non-dominant hand. I have written several stories for the grandkids and plan to write for my grown children as well.

I like to cook and entertain, although I can no longer taste food. I cook from tried-and-true recipes and memory, and it helps that my husband is a good taste-tester. It's the nurturing aspect of entertaining I find so satisfying. I try to provide a pleasant setting with flowers, candles, music and linens and then plan for conversation that engages the guest(s) and shows interest in their thoughts and opinions. For my part, I must plan on at least three times the actual time and effort I might have spent on such an occasion another lifetime ago.

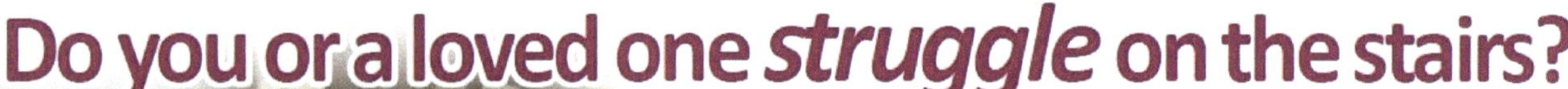

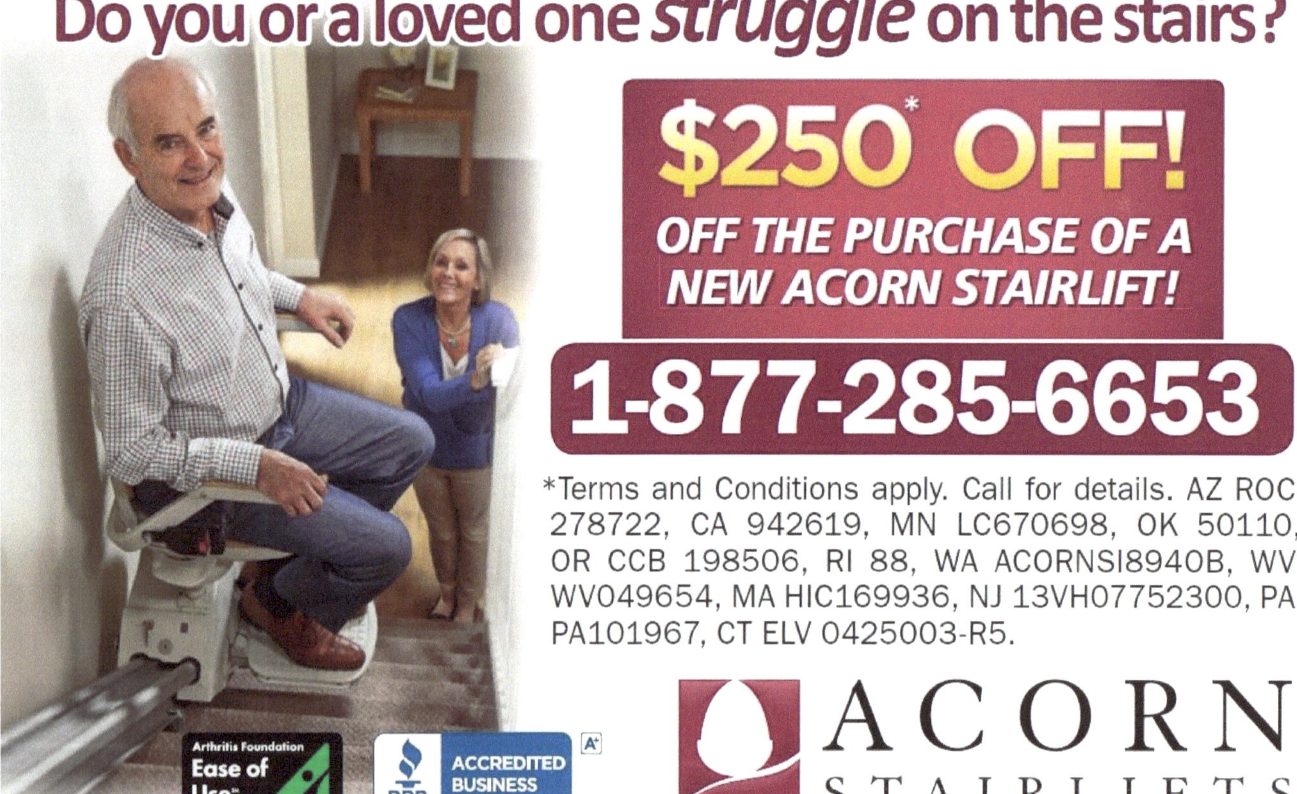

As much as I enjoy people, I have trouble thus far striking a balance between the right amount of hustle and too much. I fatigue easily and profoundly, so I need to care for my rest needs. I must become better at recognizing the need for rest, and then be disciplined enough to go lie down.

I think the most significant thing I've learned post brain injury is that life goes on—provided life goes on. One can be happy again. Many years ago, I was given a book entitled *Happiness is a Choice*. I don't think I ever read the book, but the title stuck with me. I find it to be true: happiness IS a choice. I CHOOSE to be happy. I wasn't always able to make that choice.

There was a point in time when I was so disappointed and so hurt, that I seriously contemplated going to bed and waiting to die. I had a decision to make.

I could give up or go on. Something told me, an inner voice, that there is purpose in all of this. The best is yet to come if I will do my part: be available, be hopeful, have faith. And practice gratitude. I find much to be thankful for each day, which helps my attitude.

As of today, I have done the hard work that allows me to say I'm happy. I have grieved my losses. Sometimes I still grieve, but more often than not, I feel gratitude for the people in my life, the abilities I still possess as of this moment, and more than anything I'm grateful to give and receive love.

I think I'm better at both the giving and receiving of it since the brain injury.

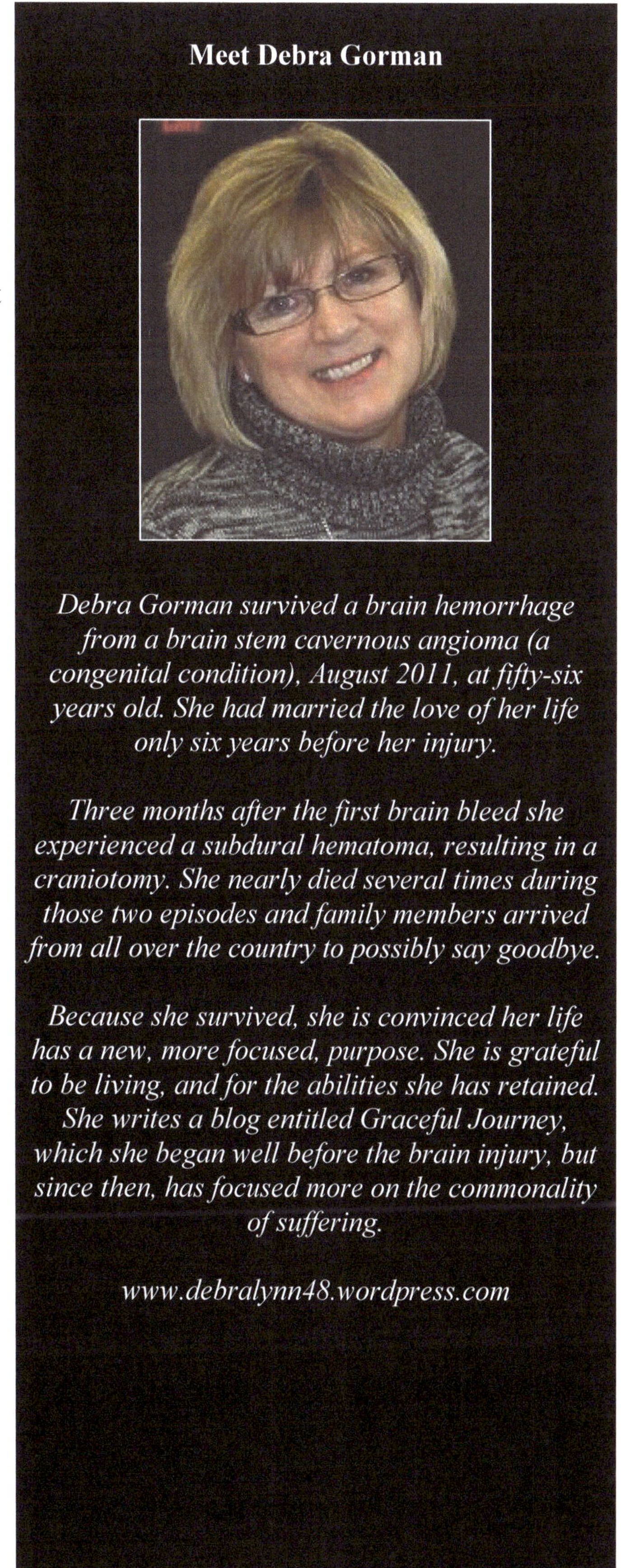

Meet Debra Gorman

Debra Gorman survived a brain hemorrhage from a brain stem cavernous angioma (a congenital condition), August 2011, at fifty-six years old. She had married the love of her life only six years before her injury.

Three months after the first brain bleed she experienced a subdural hematoma, resulting in a craniotomy. She nearly died several times during those two episodes and family members arrived from all over the country to possibly say goodbye.

Because she survived, she is convinced her life has a new, more focused, purpose. She is grateful to be living, and for the abilities she has retained. She writes a blog entitled Graceful Journey, which she began well before the brain injury, but since then, has focused more on the commonality of suffering.

www.debralynn48.wordpress.com

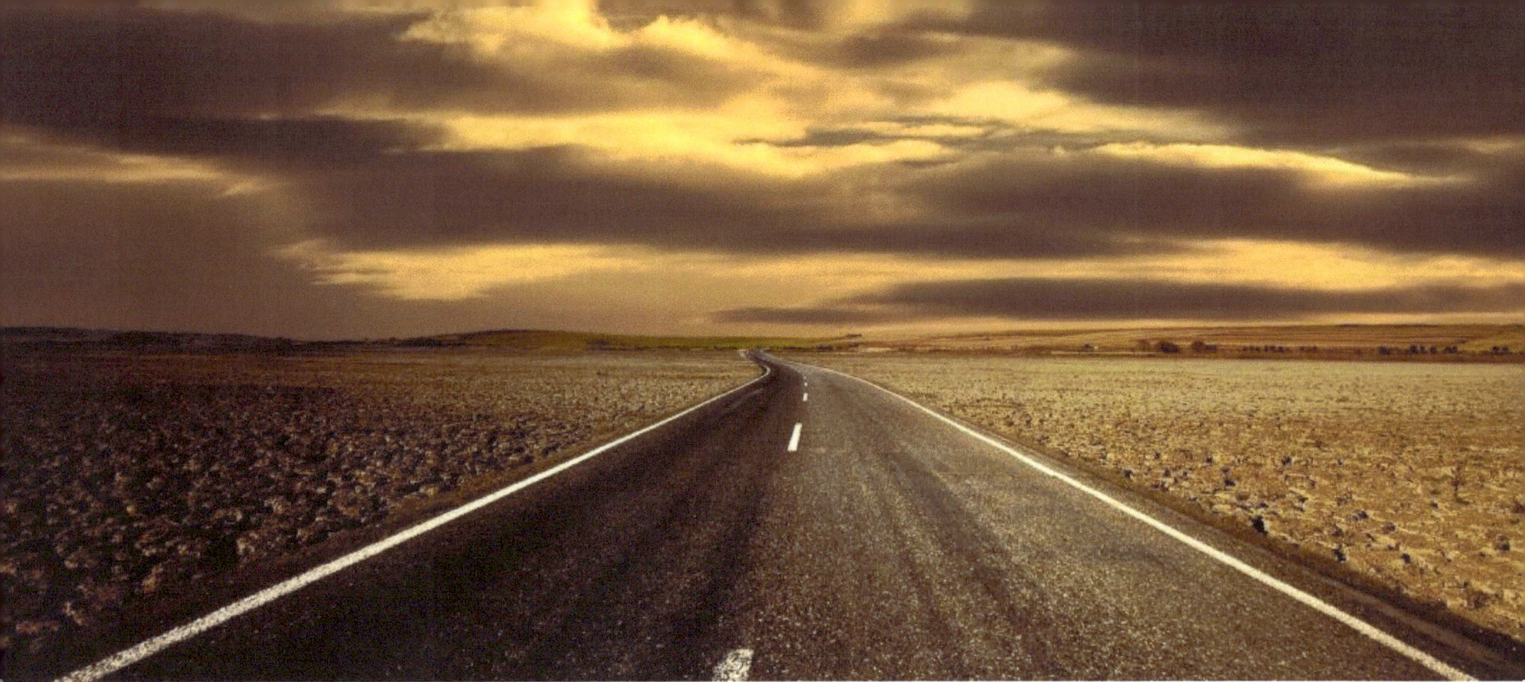

The Long Road to Recovery
By Nicole Charisi

Grace Pannell remembers the day the doctors said she would never hold a job or attend college, how they told her parents to make arrangements for her to live at home for the rest of her life.

But Pannell, now a senior special education major at Winthrop University, never lost her faith.

"The doctors said that the brain was not healing, and at this point, the greatest amounts of healing should have already happened," she recalled.

Six months earlier, Pannell jumped for a rebound while playing basketball. Her feet were swept from under her, and the back of her head hit the floor, not once, but twice. Through intense pain, Pannell got to her feet, but the world appeared blurry and uneven, and she fell several more times. Unbeknownst to her, she had already entered the game with a concussion. The damage was done.

The rest of the year was a blur of CT scans, doctors' visits, MRIs/MRAs, and monitoring. She slept on a mattress on the living room floor, always watched by a parent or her little sister. She had forgotten how to read, could barely communicate, and suffered a constant searing headache. Her parents converted the basement into an apartment for her, thinking she would live with them permanently. Then, doctors found the true cause of her pain: a misdiagnosed brain bleed, resulting in a traumatic brain injury (TBI).

"I remember hearing this and considering what it meant for my life," she said. "I remember thinking that if this is what God had for me, then I would be content. But if in any way at all He had another plan, I was trusting He would make His plan happen for my life. I found peace, hope and comfort in knowing that He was able to do anything He desired and that He had not and would not ever lose control."

Through the long road to recovery, Pannell always turned to her faith and found comfort in thinking about God's plan for her life.

Eighteen months after her injury, she woke up and just felt "different."

"My head hurt, but it was not the constant pain that I had before," she said. "I felt like I had slept that night, which was new because I always felt like I had stayed up all night. That day was the start to coming back to 'regular' life."

Six months later, she enrolled at Winthrop. She joined Cross Impact and the Baptist Collegiate Ministry (BCM), worked as a peer mentor, and volunteers with Harvest Baptist of Rock Hill. During the week, she also volunteers at a psychiatric treatment center, where she works with young girls and provides religious counseling. During the summers, she works as a camp counselor.

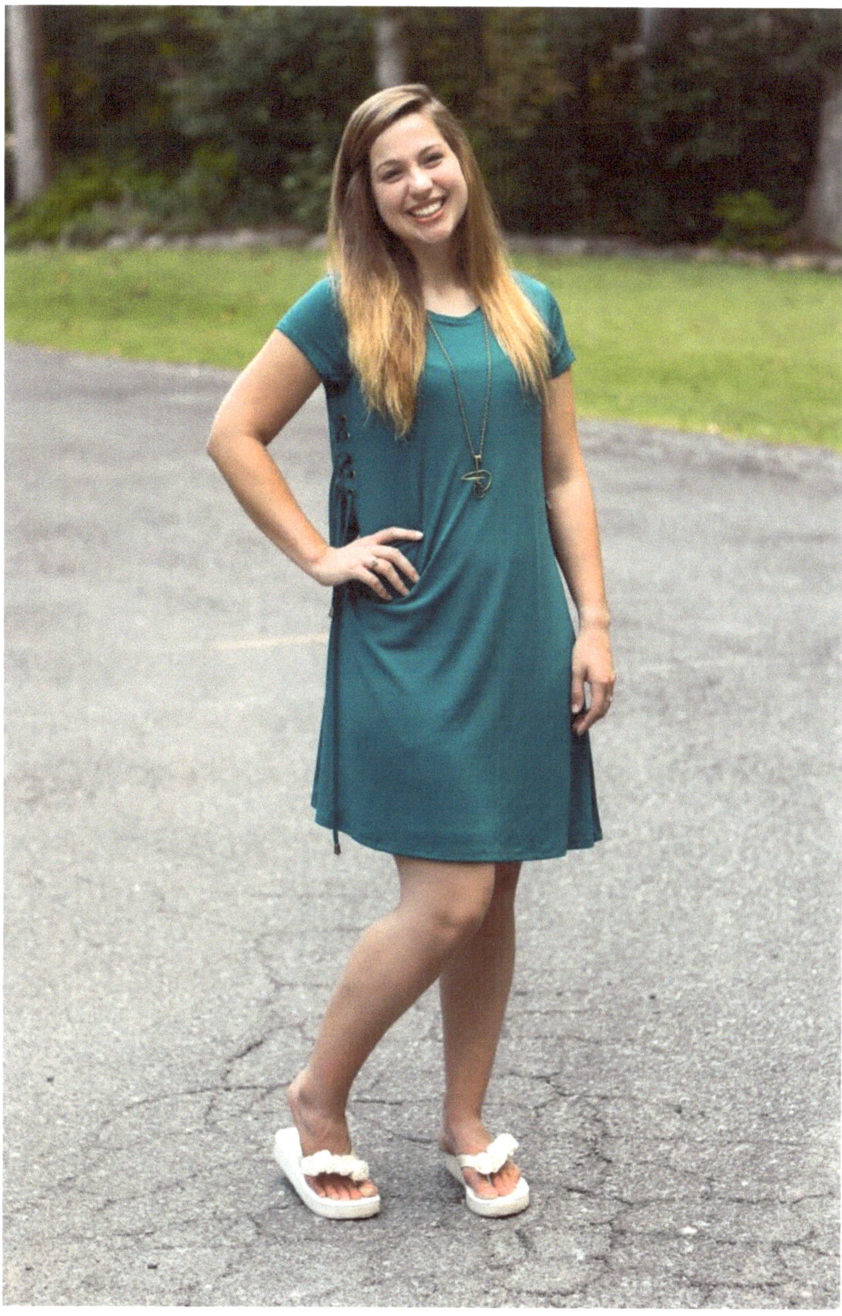

Grace Pannell Today. Photo courtesy of Blonde Moments Photography

Pannell believes going through her TBI experience, one which she still endures every day, will make her a better and more understanding teacher in the classroom, particularly with those who have special needs. She calls her TBI one of "the greatest gifts I've ever been given."

"I remember what it was like to not be able to express what I was thinking," she said. "I want to be kind and loving as I meet the needs of those whose brains work just a little differently than most. They are not less than anyone else; they simply have a brain that works a little differently than others. For a while, my brain worked differently too, so I understand in a small way what it is like."

She goes on, "And these struggles are also nothing compared to what some people carry each and every day. We all have hurts that go unseen; mine just happens to be a brain injury. But with a good, loving, perfect and powerful God I know that He is working this for good and He will continue the work that He has started."

Meet Nicole Charisi

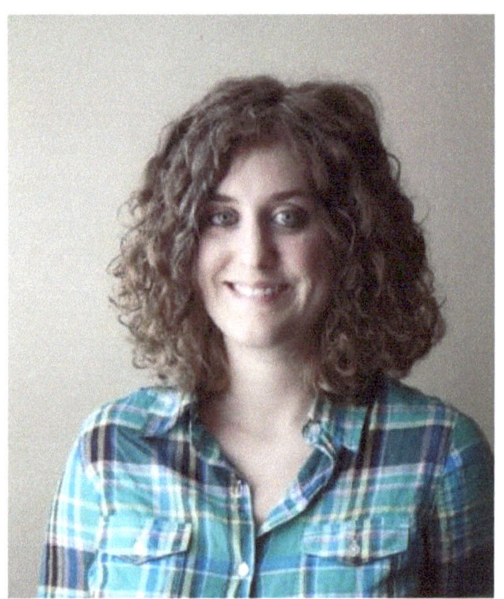

Nicole Chisari is the communications coordinator for Winthrop University in Rock Hill, South Carolina.

She holds a Bachelor of Arts in Mass Communication and a Master of Liberal Arts, both from Winthrop. She loves social media, books, and her one-year-old son.

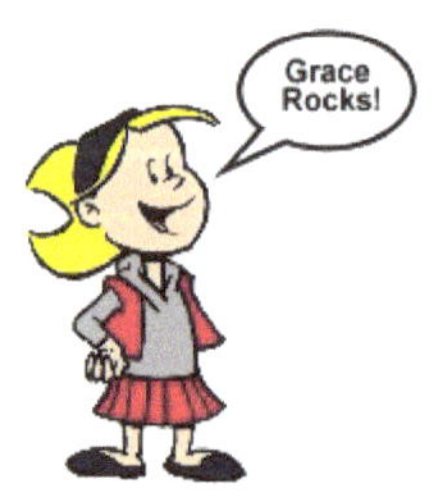

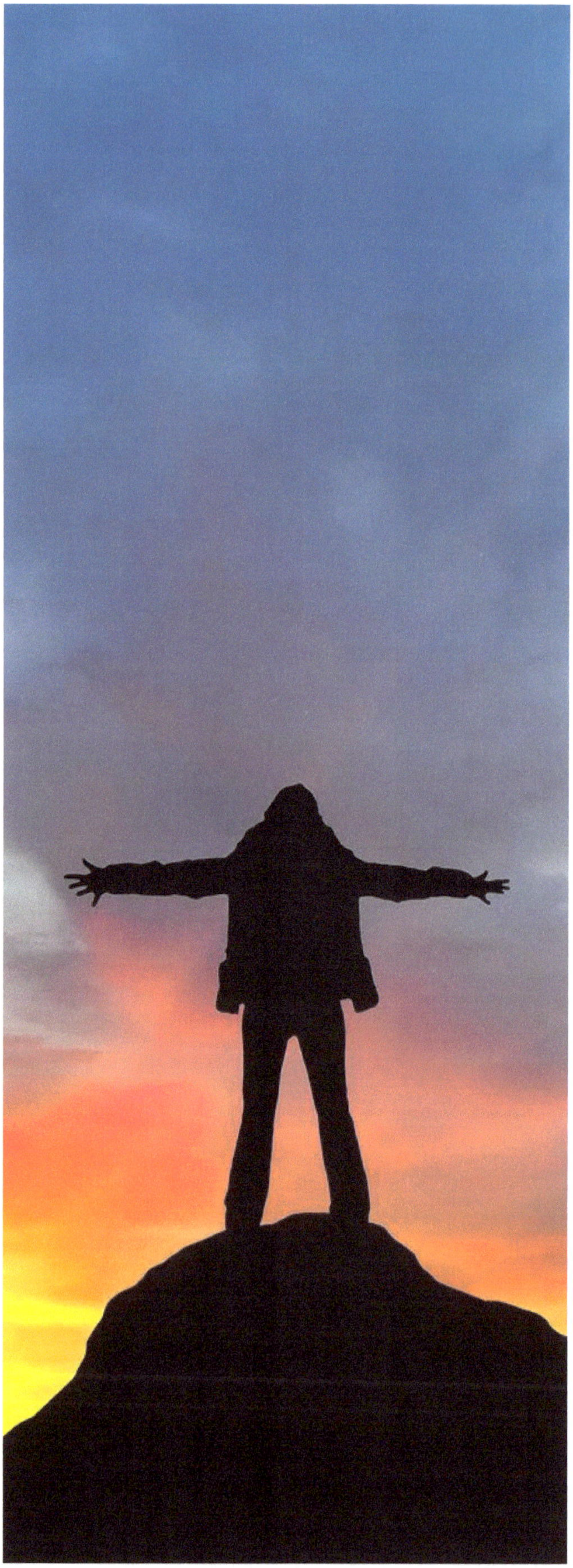

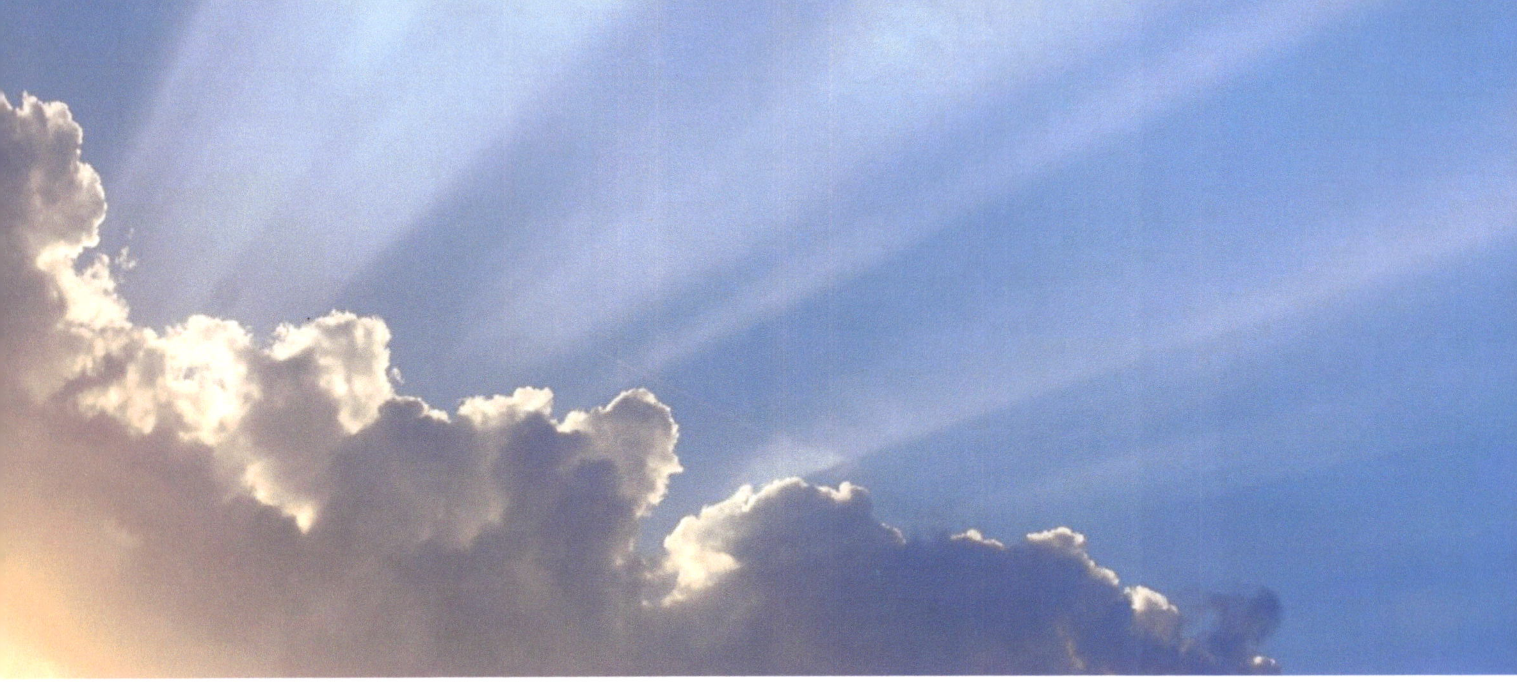

Postcards from God

By Doug Prunier

On Sept 10, 2016 my parents, my son, and I were on our way to a restaurant to celebrate the end of a successful day and the completion of a renovation project. We were stopped at a traffic light in front of the mall just blocks from our destination when a car plowed into us from behind at full city speed. The driver of the other car had over thirty years of driving experience and was picking his kids up from that very same mall. My dad, who was driving the car we were in, saw the driver behind us approaching with one hand on the wheel and staring down at his lap, but not in enough time to warn us of the imminent collision.

Fortunately, my parents, my son, and the other driver were just shaken up but not injured. Because of the way my body hit the seat and headrest, I suffered a TBI. The area that controls all the muscles on the left side of my body is the area of the brain that is most affected. While not a complete loss, it's severely limited. I have spent the last year learning how to walk and use my left arm with very little change to show for it. At the time of the accident I was an avid outdoorsman and private pilot.

> **Because of the way my body hit the seat and headrest, I suffered a TBI.**

The accident doesn't define who I am now. I'm still a husband and father of 5, but it absolutely defines what I can still do. There is not a single aspect of my daily activities that is not limited by the injury. But more painful than that for me is that everything is tainted with all of the memories from my past accomplishments before the accident as well. The reality of the accident is so ingrained (if even just under the surface,) that every time I'm about to share something on social media that's happy, funny, or

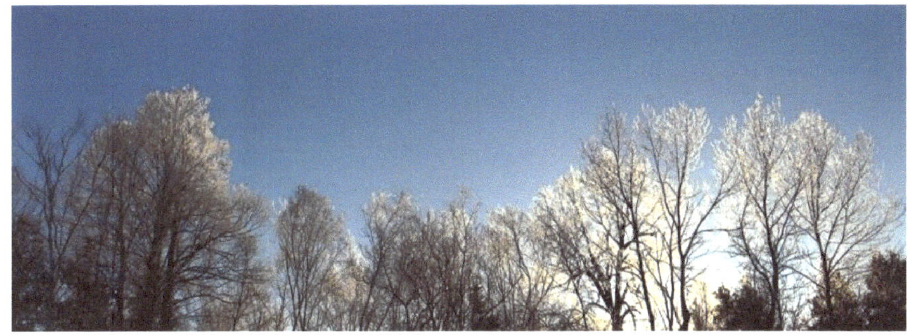

beautiful, I feel that I'm lying by omission because there is a significant part of the story that I'm not telling, and in most cases that keeps me from sharing all together.

In fact I have wanted to change my cover photo on Facebook for several months, but I can't get away from the fact that it most accurately reflects my post-accident reality even one year later. All signs of life in my hopes and dreams that I had before the accident are now dormant and look dead, frozen in time and covered in frost that signals the beginning of the long winter ahead. But more importantly, even in the shadow of this frozen waste land, I can see the reflections of light and the hope of a distant spring. Even though I can't see the sun at this moment, I can see evidence of its existence just beyond the horizon. All I can do now is patiently wait for spring while wondering what will survive the harsh winter ahead.

The only reason I wanted to share about the pain (physical but mostly emotional) was to share how I experienced love of God in that pain.

After the TBI, the advice from the doctors was "sit quiet and let your brain heal." We live out in the country and get only three channels on the television, and internet service is not much better, so I had to find something else to do. I started sitting under the bird feeder with my camera to get good reference photos of the song birds in our yard. I became such a natural part of the landscape that the birds would routinely land on me, even with a cat on my lap.

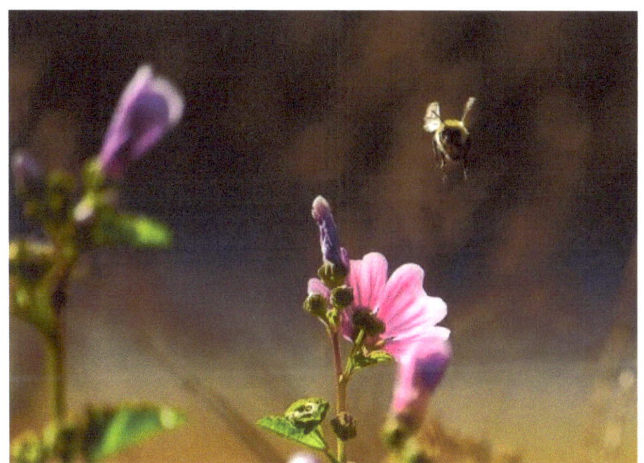

One day when there was not much bird action, I snapped a shot of a bumble bee near a flower in our weed infested and overgrown flower bed for no other reason than sheer boredom; no setup, just a reflex. Afterwards, I spent days just staring at the picture that turned out because the contrast between what I was feeling in my heart at the time and the beauty in the photo was just too great for me to ignore. This was only a small sample of the world around me for the duration of 1/1000th of a second and it was breathtaking, for me in that moment at least. This photo was taken less than two weeks after the accident.

This went on for months. I was crying on the inside while pressing the shutter button, and then being totally surprised because I could see instantly the beauty of God around me. I was in the midst of the biggest storm in my life, but my best photos are capturing the essence of calm and tranquility. I had no choice but to admit that God really is in my suffering because the emotion that was being conveyed in my photos was not coming from me. I really felt God answering my prayers one photo at a time. Some of my "Best of 2016" collection were taken just nine days after the accident.

For me, these photos were always more than just pretty pictures, but captures of moments of the ongoing work of the Real Artist always at work around us but, it took looking through my camera lens to see it. One year later, I still struggle to see the beauty in the world around me without the aid of the camera, but at the same time my camera has also become my most effective pain reliever. It means so much to me when I hear that my photos captured a special moment for someone else as well but I will always see them as postcards from God.

Meet Doug Prunier

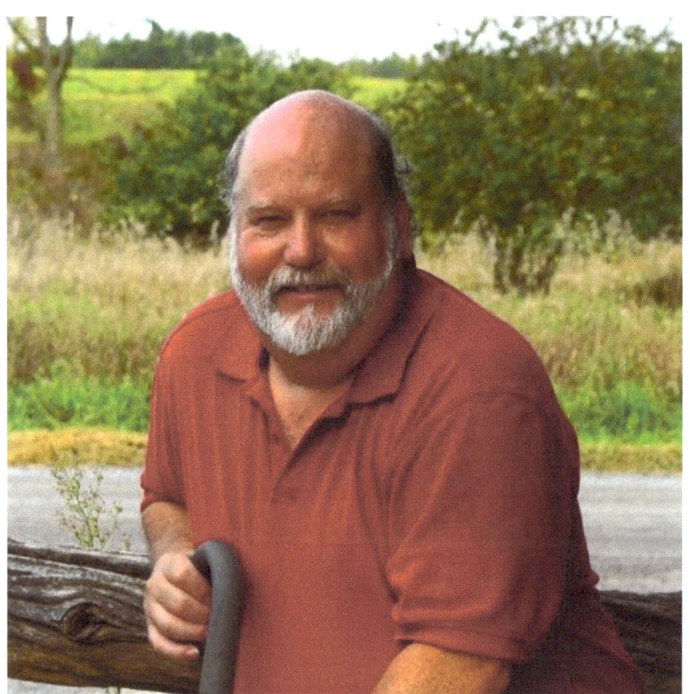

Doug writes…

I just turned fifty and I am a husband and a father to five kids age eight to twenty-one. I live near Ottawa Ontario Canada. I transitioned to a stay-at-home dad nineteen years ago from the high tech industry to have a more active role in my kids' lives. From a very young age we enjoyed many adventures such as; "arts & crafts with dad" which involved power tools, 30+ mile day trips by bicycle and flying and maintaining our small airplane.

On September 10, 2016, I was rear ended by a distracted driver and lost significant use of my left side as a result of a TBI. I have spent the last year learning to walk and my youngest now gets to teach me how to catch a ball!

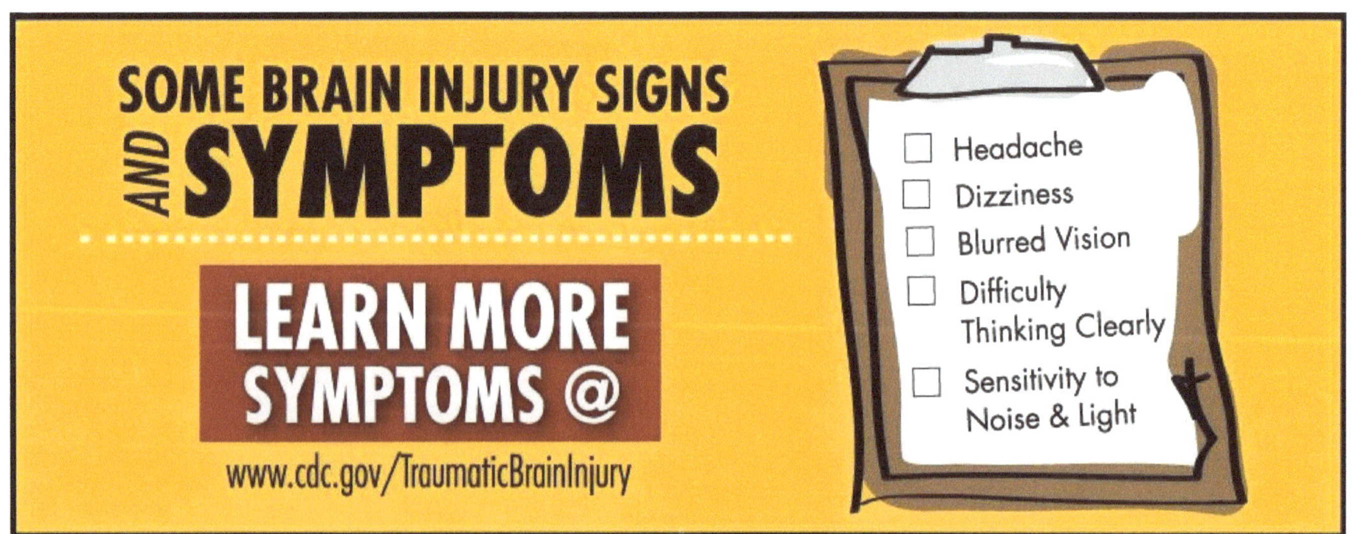

News & Views

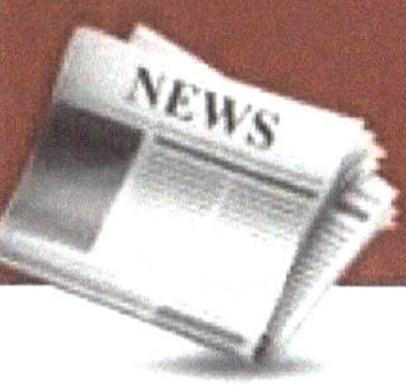

Rarely a week goes by these days that I do not hear about concussion in the news. This is very different from the way things were seven short years ago when I sustained my own traumatic brain injury. A few weeks ago, I heard a rather telling story on a local radio station. It seems that a local town had a "Twelve-years-old and under" football league for many years. The local community cancelled the league this year for an interesting reason – lack of participation.

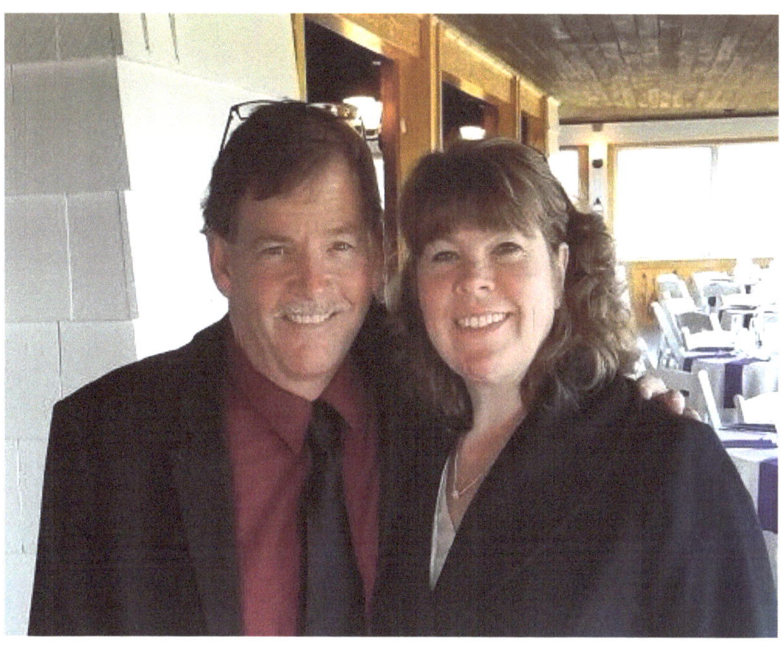

Where there had been hundreds of participants in years past, this year only a dozen kids expressed interest in playing and the league was subsequently cancelled.

I will not use this space to share my opinion about ANY sport that can leave participants compromised for life, Rather I view this as a dramatic swing in both public opinion about the dangers of impact sports and a direct reflection of how the general public is now making choices based on an increased level of exposure via the mainstream media.

Ever the realist, I know that we will never live in a world without risk. But as time passes, it is my hope that fewer and fewer people will be in the position of having to live with all that comes with living daily with a brain injury.

Seen in this light, it feels good to see that forward progress is indeed being made.

Until next month,

~David & Sarah Grant